INTUITIVE EATING

How you can feel free from chronic dieting with this healthy revolutionary way that works for weight loss without keto diet or intermittent fasting. honor your hunger.

Catherine Silas

TABLE OF CONTENTS

INTUITIVE EATING

WORKBOOK

Stop Keto Diet Or Intermittent Fasting With A
Step By Step Mindful Based Program For
Weight Loss, Design Your Body Image And
Have A Healthy Relationship With Food.

Catherine Silas

TABLE OF CONTENTS

INTRODUCTION

This book is not a diet book. It does not tell you what you should eat, what you shouldn't eat, when to eat and when not to eat. This book is for people who have gone through so many diets and eating plans and have found that nothing has worked. This book is here to help you reclaim your connection with food and make peace with it.

While you go through this book, you will learn about best practices concerning your relationship with food, you'll also find information on food types, low carb foods, superfoods, you will also read about water fasting and even intermittent fasting. This information is written in this book to help you seek what is best for you in nurturing your body rather than go through starvation. It also encourages natural weight loss based on what good feels like for you, helping you find the weight that you were meant to be in. Overall it helps you achieve a renewed sense of understanding about food. Before you begin, here are 10 principles to remind you about intuitive eating:

1. Reject the diet mentality

Diets and eating plans have been created to help plenty of people out there meet their weight loss goals. The problem with diets and us is that we have already created a bad relationship with food and when we attempt a diet, we fail because we put too much hope and went all in too fast and unsatisfactory results. This perception itself prevents you from rediscovering intuitive eating.

2. Honor your hunger

As you read this book, you will come to learn how to honor your hunger and how to keep your body biologically fed with adequate nutrition. We will discuss overeating, how to stop overeating as well as learning to honor the first signals of satiety.

3. Make peace with food

A large part of intuitive eating is to make peace with food and work on creating a relationship that prevents you from feeling deprived which could cause binge eating and cravings. It is to help you understand why you eat the way you eat and how you can change your eating habits to better ones.

4. Challenge our Food Police

There will be plenty of thoughts running through your mind when you indulge or when you just have a simple meal. These are all unreasonable rules we pick up along the way as we grow, identifying certain foods as 'bad' and certain foods as 'good'. Through intuitive eating, you will learn to change this critical step and make mindful decisions of your food choices.

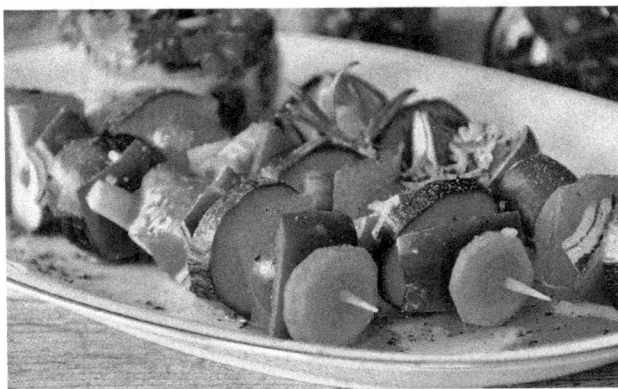

5. Respecting your Satiety

We will also learn how to listen to our bodies for signals when it tells you that you are no longer hungry. You will also learn to observe and honor these signs and learn to eat through not only your mouth but through other senses from sight, smell and touch.

6. Discover your Satisfaction Factor

One of the most basic gifts to humankind is the pleasure and satisfaction of eating experiences. When we eat what we really want to it, the pleasure you derive is a powerful force that helps you feel satisfied and content. Why allowing yourself to feel happy and satisfied in your meal, you will notice that it takes much less food to feel pleasure.

7. Honor your feelings without food

Many of us use food as a way to comfort ourselves when we feel emotions especially negative emotions from anxiety, boredom, loneliness as well as anger. One of the objectives of intuitive eating is to remove this emotional aspect away from food and to make us more aware of our food triggers. We will learn that food can only provide temporary relief and that it will not fix any of these feelings. If anything, emotional eating only makes you feel guilty. By honoring our emotions without food, we respect both our feelings and the food we consume.

8. Respect our body

Intuitive eating helps you accept your genetic blueprint. Each of us has different body compositions and it is unrealistic to think that humans all come in one size. By understanding this, we all remove unrealistic expectations of how our bodies should look. More than that, we also respect our body so you can also feel better about who you are and prevent yourself from being critical about your body shape.

9. Exercising

Exercise is crucial but that does not mean you must spend more than an hour in the gym or go through an intensive boot camp to get the body you want. Exercising here is just to get active, to move and feel different. Exercising comes in all shapes and forms and it is more about shifting your focus from how many calories you burn to how you feel from working out, the energy you feel. Exercising can be anything from a brisk walk to a stroll in the park to a 30 minute HIIT workout.

10. Honor your Health

Last but not least, intuitive eating also enables you to look at food as fuel and not just as a means to an end for your hunger. You will be geared to make better food choices that honor your taste buds as well as your health and that does not mean it must come out from a perfect nutrition diet. You will not suffer a nutrient deficiency or gain weight if you eat a slice of pizza or if you had a brownie. Intuitive eating helps you to look at eating healthily more consistently and that progress, and not perfection is what is important.

CHAPTER 1-

UNDERSTANDING INTUITIVE EATING

There's a pretty good reason why you decided to choose this book to read. It could be because you are tired with all the various diets you took on and still did not meet your desired weight or it could be that you tried to eat healthily but failed at some point because there were too many distractions. It could also be you tried eating routines such as intermittent fasting to regulate your eating patterns but it did not work out. Whatever your reasons may be, considering a better relationship with food will help you eat well and have a better focus on weight loss as well as health.

What is Intuitive Eating?

Intuitive eating a method of eating. It focuses on you being the expert of your body as well as your body's hunger signals. It is not a traditional diet. There are no guidelines for what you should eat or what you should not eat and no guidelines to when you should be eating.

With intuitive eating, you are the sole focus, the only person that makes choices of the food that goes into your mouth. It teaches you that you are the best person to make all these food choices.

What Are the basics of Intuitive Eating?

Intuitive eating promotes a healthy attitude towards body image and its relationship with food. The idea with intuitive eating is that you should eat only when you are hungry and stop when you are full. Sounds simple? The hardest part is making that choice. It is that intuitive process where you remind yourself that you are the person that will make that choice- you put yourself first and as the primary decision-maker of your life and your body.

To eat intuitively, the first thing to do is to re-learn to trust your body and to make this intuitive process easier and for that to take place, you need to distinguish the difference between physical hunger and emotional hunger

Physical hunger- This is a biological need to replenish the nutrients in your body. This kind of hunger builds gradually and it has different signals such as fatigue, growling stomach as well as irritability. You are only satisfied when you have eaten some food. Emotional hunger- This type of hunger is emotionally driven. It stems from boredom or loneliness and even sadness and other feelings that could trigger cravings for food This type of hunger creates self-hatred as well as guilt.

How Did Intuitive Eating Begin?

First coined in 1995 by Evelyn Tribole and Elyse Resch as the title of their book, this concept however begins earlier on through other philosophies. The earlier ideations came from Susie Orbach, the author of 'Fat is a Feminist Issue' back in 1978. Before that, Geneen Roth also explored this concept when writing about emotional eating in 1982.

The thought process of intuitive eating was built on the foundation that diets or eating plans do not work and it is about a lifestyle change that focuses on personal care for more sustainable weight loss.

The Research and Benefits Behind Intuitive Eating

The research on intuitive eating is still growing and for the moment, most of it is focused on women. However, all research conducted so far has shown that intuitive eating leads to healthier psychological behaviors, better weight maintenance as well as lower body mass index. Per the National Center for Biotechnology Information, the major benefit of intuitive eating is that it leads to psychological health. Participants for intuitive eating research has shown improved self-esteem, overall quality of life as well as better image.

Research published in Science Direct also says that intuitive eating provides better retention rates which means those going through this method have a better chance of sticking to the program and practice mindful changes than they would if they were on a diet. Studies focused on women's eating behaviors and their attitudes show that women who intuitively eat are less likely to display behaviors related to eating disorders.

1.1 What Is Overeating?

Overeating refers to the behavior of eating more calories than the body uses for energy. In other words, people who overeat usually do it for psychological or emotional reasons such as anxiety, depression, boredom as well as stress. Not sure if you are eating too much? Well, one way to figure this out would be to review your accurate or correct amount of daily calories that your body needs depending on your age, metabolism as well as current weight and level of physical activity as well as gender. For example, a woman who is 150 pounds and works out regularly would require more calories than a woman of the same size but does not exercise regularly. The <u>Dietary Guidelines for Americans</u> would be a good source of information regarding the right amount based on your body type and level of fitness. Overeating leads to various health problems, the chief of call obesity, high blood pressure, heart diseases as well as high cholesterol. This is the main reason why you need to keep your food portions under control.

Are there signs of eating too much?

One of the main ways to understand or to identify if you have eaten too much is to ask yourself how you feel once you have eaten. Do you feel bloated or uncomfortable? Do you feel gassy or discomfort? These may all be major signs of overeating. If you overeat, you may also feel distressed or embarrassed once you are done with your meal. Those who overeat usually feel like they have less control over how much and what they consume.

Having no success in diets could also be a major indication that you struggle with overeating. Another aspect of overeating could also indicate BED or binge eating disorder. Among the primary signs of BED are eating until you feel uncomfortably full or eating faster than normal, consuming large amounts of food even when you are not hungry as well as eating alone all the time. If you notice that you have eaten too much (and doing this often) you should work with your dietitian or your doctor to create a healthy meal plan for you.

Is there a way to stop overeating?

Once you have answered the question about whether you are overeating, your next step is to act. These actions are the first few steps towards keeping track of what you eat and how much or even when you eat. It requires you to be disciplined to record your meals, snacks, and drinks to help manage your food portions. The **National Institute of Diabetes and Digestive and Kidney Diseases** (NIDDKD) recommends that the best way to track what goes into your diet is by making it a habit to check food labels so you can see what goes into the process of creating that particular meal or food item as well as the number of calories per serving.

All of this can be included in a food tracker (there's an app for that for your phone) or you can also input this into your online calendar or do it the manual way which is to write this into your notebook. Once you start tracking your food intake, you'd be surprised to find out the details of your eating habits well as make yourself accountable for what you eat and your progress towards better eating. The NIDDKD offers these tips for managing your food portions at home:

- Eating only one serving based on the food label or recipe

- Eating your food slowly to allow your brain to receive signals that your stomach is full

- Exchanging larger plates and glasses with smaller ones to help you eat less and drink less

- Fill your plate mostly with low-calorie foods or foods that are low in saturated fats

- Eating your meals at the same time every day

- Never skipping meals as it could lead to overeating

You also need to watch your portions when eating out and especially at buffets. When eating out or in buffets, make healthier and lighter food choices. It is also easy to overeat when we watch TV and if you do this, the Center for Disease Control and Prevention recommends that you either snack on healthier options or place snacks in containers so you can eat only a certain amount. Try not to snack straight out of the package.

1.2. Food and weight loss

In the United States, more than 2 in 3 adults are either obese or overweight. The fact that you're overweight also means that it has a high probability of leading to plenty of diseases that affect women (and also men) such as diabetes, heart diseases as well as certain types of cancer. Talking about your weight can be uncomfortable to plenty of people but if you find a medical practitioner such as a doctor or a nurse that you are comfortable with, they can be a valuable partner in your journey to lose weight.

How would you know if you are obese or overweight?

Apart from the physical aspects which are the most obvious signs, another good indicator is to look at our Body Mass Index (BMI). This index can be used to determine if your weight is in a healthy range with your height. This tool helps to estimate your body fat and you use your height x weight into the BMI calculator created by the Centers for Disease Control and Prevention.

This BMI indicator just gives you an indication of how healthy your weight is. However, this does not by any means count as accurate. The BMI count is less accurate for some people compared to others. For instance, for muscular people, their BMI may be above 25 because muscle weigh more than fat.

Another good way to understand the healthiness of your weight is by looking at your waist circumference. Weight researchers and doctors agree that women with a circumference of their waist larger than 35 inches are considered overweight or obese.

What is the cause of obesity?

A person becomes obese when their body ends up storing more calories than it uses. Your body does need calories such as minerals, essential vitamins, and nutrients for it to remain healthy and active. If your body uses less of these calories than it stores, this will cause you to gain weight.

Other causes can also be a person's environment over a lifetime that can cause obesity. This is in relation to the food you eat but it could also be influenced by other factors that are not within your control such as availability of healthy food, pollution or even access to safe places to exercise, gyms or even parks.

How common are obesity and overweight?

At least where the United States is concerned, it is very common. Women of all races, ages, and ethnicities can be obese and overweight however, in some groups, overweight and obesity are more prevalent. Apart from food and external factors, there are other factors that cause obesity which are things like family background and event past events as well as the place where you live.

If you find it hard to exercise or incorporate any kind of physical activity or you are worried about your weight, you can speak to a doctor or dietician. Also, there could be some risk factors that cause obesity and overweight that are beyond your control. Your dietician, doctor or nurse would be able to recommend healthier eating habits as well as exercises to help you reach a more optimal weight. Also, there could be some medication that could cause weight gain so this is something you need to tell your doctor if you are in the process of changing the way you eat and live.

What individual factors unique to me can make it more likely that I'll gain weight? Obesity affects a person in many ways, and this can happen over a long period of time. The factors that influence our weight are such as:

Our family background and genes- There is not just one 'fat' gene. Obesity runs in families and there are different genes that work to make a person more likely to gain weight. The situation that you are in also affects your genes and this could have begun at infancy based on the eating and physical activity instilled in you by your parents or caregiver when you were a child.

Your Metabolism- some people are blessed with very good metabolism. Metabolism is the ability of your body to burn calories and this affects your weight gain or weight loss. Men who are muscular for instance burn more calories quickly. Women's metabolism might change throughout their lives depending on changes that take place during puberty, pregnancy as well as menopause.

Your Age- Of course, your metabolism gets slower the older you get. We also tend to lose muscle as we age, and the less muscle means we burn calories less.

Any trauma- the traumatic events that have taken place in our lives are something that we may not have control over, and this can cause either weight gain or weight loss. Women (and yes men too) who experience negative events during childhood, such as abuse, parental divorce, road accidents can lead to obesity in adults. Girls who are sexually abused, research has pointed out, are more likely to gain weight when they become adults and eventually lead to obesity. Those that experience PTSD also are highly likely to gain weight as well.

Medication could also lead to weight gain. Medicines related to sleep, mental health can lead to weight gain or it could also make it difficult to lose weight. If you are taking any prescriptions that may cause you to put on weight or make it difficult to lose weight, you should let your doctor know about it.

Not Getting Enough Sleep can also cause weight gain simply because it affects your hormone levels and that affects your food choices as well as your appetite. Not being well-rested also affects whether you have the energy for exercise throughout the day.

How can the location of where I live make it more likely that I'll gain weight?

The surroundings in which we live may be a cause of weight gain in people. These things are such as:

- • **Your neighborhood**- Look around you and see how safe or easy it is for you to exercise? Some neighborhoods that do not have parks or sidewalks or even a gym nearby that makes it difficult to do even simple physical activities such as brisk walking or running. There could be traffic or even safety issues with even taking your dog out for a walk. Some places can also be unsafe for those with disabilities too.

- • **Your access to healthy food**- Our access to healthy food also influences our weight gain. Healthy food can be expensive and many people do not have the luxury of low-cost healthy options for food at the places where they live. It could also be that your route to and fro from work or school has most fast-food restaurants than access to a grocery store where you can get fresh produce.

- • **Pollution in your area**- Things like secondhand smoke, air pollution (like haze) is also linked to obesity. Chemicals also exist in the food we eat so if there's pollution, there is also a likelihood that it has permeated into your food too and this leads to obesity.

1.3. Benefits of mindful eating

What benefits should a balanced and healthy body bring me?

A healthy individual is one who also has a clean bill of health. If you haven't had a regular or recent check-up with your local GP, you should get one before you begin the intermittent fasting method. An individual with a clean bill of health is at a lower risk of contracting any deadly diseases which include cardiovascular problems, diabetes, arthritis and more. This is what you should strive to be. Exercising regularly is something that you need to start doing if you're not already doing it. If you want to be healthy, exercise is going to have to be a part of that package. Not only does it help to regulate your body's blood flow, but it also helps to balance out and boost your metabolism, which goes without saying is needed for overall good health.

When you are in good health and you are eating right it shows both physically and you also feel it internally, here is what's going to happen:

You Become a More Confident Person – Living a healthy lifestyle can do wonders for your mental and emotional health. You're going to start feeling really good about yourself because you like the results that you see in the mirror. A healthy diet and regular exercise will give your body that healthy look and glow that no cosmetic product or makeup would ever replicate because that glow is going to come from within. When you know that you look good, you start to feel good. You're energetic, you're clear-minded, you feel good, and you feel like you are ready to take on any challenge that is thrust at you. You become a more confident person.

You're Emotionally More Stable – Our emotional state is linked to good health because believe it or not, the mood is psychosomatic. When your body does not feel good, don't expect your mind to be feeling all that great either. Mood swings will become inevitable when a person experiences hormonal ups and downs as a result of poor health. If you find this hard to believe, just think of a time when you came down with a cold and felt fantastic emotionally. Almost certainly the answer is going to be *never* because it is impossible for us to feel any kind of happy when our bodies are not working as it should be. That is a perfect example of why good health is so important because being healthy will help your body boost its serotonin levels, which is also known as the happiness hormone. Yes, that hormone exists, why do you think you get that rush of happiness when you consume alcohol or ice cream for example? Because of the temporary spike in serotonin that you just received. What to feel that way all the time? Be healthy.

You Obviously Look Much Better – This goes without saying. Sugary drinks, fatty foods, and junk food may give you a temporary glow and feeling of happiness, but that is only going to be short-lived. Why? Because eating too much junk like that is also going to cause you wrinkles and some extra, unwanted padding around your waist. Plus, it makes you feel lethargic and sluggish when you are carrying around more weight than you should, which is what a lot of obese people feel like all the time. Being healthy and consuming enough water, getting ample sleep and eating a nutritious diet packed with fruits, vegetables, grains, protein and more is the secret to keeping your skin looking healthy and your hair shiny. Not only are you going to find that you look better, but your movements are going to become a lot more energized, which will give you an overall look for appearing more attractive, youthful and supple.

You Become More Productive – Because we can't always rely on coffee and tobacco to give us that spike in energy that we need. It's only a momentary spike and it won't last long, wouldn't you prefer having that feeling all day long? A balanced lifestyle and good health are how you achieve that same spike in energy that coffee can give you each morning. Cut down that dependency of getting your energy sources from elsewhere and instead, just choose good health to feel that way all the time.

You Don't Spend Any Extra Time – Knowing what you are eating possibly even saves you time because that 30 minutes to an hour which you spend on your meal could now be filled with other productive activities, which means you get more done during the day. You don't have to meal-prep as much when you're preparing one meal less, which also saves you time. Every little moment saved is a moment more that you could get more things done.

You're Able to Think Clearly – Admit it, there have been several occasions where you've often felt sluggish at work, especially after a big meal. Not just at work, but at home too. That's because your body is busy digesting food, which causes you to feel more lethargic, making you feel less productive and like you could sleep for several hours. Which is why mindful eating is so great for mental clarity since when your body is not too preoccupied with digesting its meals, your mind is better able to focus on the task you have at hand. If you're currently trying intermittent fasting and skipping lunch, you'll be able to see the difference for yourself, how there's no longer that sluggish, lazy feeling you get after eating. Instead, you feel focused, energized and ready to power through to 5 pm.

It Saves You Money – Eating one meal less means spending on one meal less, and that money can be redirected back into your savings account. You can even save money with groceries because the ingredients for your meals now last much longer when you're eating less than you normally would. When you look at how much you've been able to save at the end of the month just by cutting out one meal a day from your schedule, you'll be a lot more motivated to stick to this method even more than you already are.

It Helps You Lose Weight & Keep It Off – Needless to say, this is probably one of the biggest physical benefits that most people would look forward to. It's not just about losing weight, equally important is keeping the weight off for good, which is why eating mindfully is the only method that has proven to be able to do this. This goes back to the earlier point about not restricting yourself to only certain food groups and being able to eat regularly so you don't feel like you're depriving yourself in any way. The happier you feel about your diet and being able to eat the foods you like is the difference that makes intermittent fasting more effective than anything else out there.

You Become More Confident & Disciplined – When you look good, you feel good, which is why people embark on a weight loss journey, isn't it? Because they want to look like the best version of themselves. Intermittent fasting can do that for you, and not only will you end up looking and feeling much healthier, when you see how good you look in the mirror your confidence level increases. Your confidence levels will also be aided by the fact that eating intuitively has taught you to be a more disciplined individual, focused on a goal, and being able to accomplish a goal that you set out to do. You need some level of discipline to succeed even with intermittent fasting because you need to be able to say no in the face of delicious food when it's not your time to eat. Sticking to a regular eating regimen helps to build your discipline levels, and when you can do that, your confidence levels are one again elevated because you can look back and say yes, I did it!

It Reduces Your Risk of Developing Type 2 Diabetes – Losing weight makes your body more insulin sensitive, which lowers your blood sugar levels. Eating makes our bodies release insulin into the bloodstream so that it can supply our cells with the energy we need. However, those who are already pre-diabetic will already be insulin-resistant, which means their blood sugar levels remain elevated, and that's why going on the intermittent fasting method could go a long way in helping this. Fasting means your body would need to produce insulin less often because you're not consuming any food, which could help to stabilize your insulin secretion.

It Reduces Your Risk of Cardiovascular Disease – Fasting is not the same as starvation. You're not cutting yourself off from food completely, you're simply eating less. Minimizing your calories will help to minimize your risk of cardiovascular disease because by losing weight, you simultaneously reduce your blood pressure levels, lower your cholesterol and triacylglycerol levels, all of which help to keep heart disease at bay.

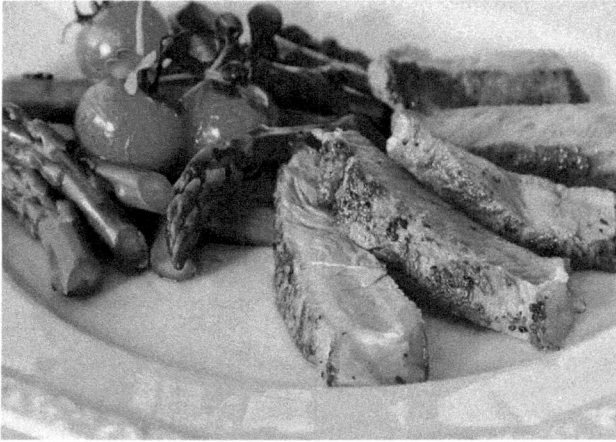

CHAPTER 2-

THE SCIENCE OF THE BRAIN AND FOOD

2.1 Your weight and food

A portion of food is how much a person chooses to eat at one time whether it is at home, in a restaurant or whether from a package. A serving refers to the amount of food listed on the product's food label or Nutritional Facts.

Different food products have different services sizes which can be measured either in pieces, in cups, in ounces, in slices, grams or even in numbers. A service size on a food label is the recommendation that should be eaten by an average adult. Depending on how much you choose to eat, your portion size may or may not equate to the serving size listed on the label.

How much should I eat?

The number of calories that you consume daily depends on whether you want to lose weight, maintain your weight, your age, your weight, your metabolic rate, your gender as well as how physically active you are. Per the Dietary Guidelines for Americans 2015-2020, you can read about it to have an idea of how many calories you would need daily based on your gender, your age, and physical fitness level.

You can also use the tools and apps to make your calories and fitness plan to help you reach and maintain your desired weight. However, the best route to go for this would be to speak to your dietitian first to get a better understanding of your body and its needs from a health care perspective.

2.2 Why we eat the way we eat?

Every person has a different relationship to food the same way all our bodies are different. There is no fixed method or equation to eat just as there is no one-size-fits all kind of body. Based on our genetics, the place we live in, our metabolism as well as our preferences. It all influences what we eat and why we eat it. While some of us graze certain food items, some of us gorge. While some of us snack, others can be comfort eating. Some people under eat while some people overeat. Some are obsessed with only raw foods while some are only vegan. Some could be pescatarians whereas some are meat-eaters through and through. Knowing yourself, who you are, what you have the most access to is one step towards intuitive eating.

How can I manage food portions at home?

You do not necessarily have to measure and count everything you eat and drink- this can be exhausting to do daily. That said, it is recommended that you train yourself to read labels and count calories for an adequate amount of time to learn and get used to the average serving and portion sizes. When eating at home, here is what you can do:

- Take one serving as recommended by the food label and eat it off a plate instead of directly out of the box or packaging.

- Try as much as possible to not eat in front of the TV, or when you are busy doing other activities like working on your computer, writing or even studying. Pay attention to the foods you eat. Keep your focus on eating, chew your food well and immerse yourself in the experience of the taste of the food

- Chew your food slowly so that you can give your brain enough time to get the message that your stomach is full. This usually takes about 15 minutes

- Eat out of smaller bowls and plates and drink out of smaller glasses so that you train your body to eat per the size of your crockery

- Minimize your consumption of chips, dips, sauces, and snacks

- Freeze food that you will not eat right away or serve right away, especially if you have made too much. Or you can also meal prep them for next day's meals.

- Keep your eating times regular every day and do not skip meals.

- If snacking, look for low-calorie choices and single-serving snacks. If you do buy big box snacks, divide them together with your meal prep so you are not tempted to overeat.

How can I manage portions when eating out?

It is easier to portion control when you are home but when eating out, it can be a little harder. If you find yourself eating out often, here are some tips that you can try to keep your food portions in check:

- Try meal prepping to avoid eating out. Meal prepping lunch for work will make it easier for you to each lunch that has been home-cooked and prevent you from eating out

- Compare the money you save eating home-made lunches versus eating out for lunch every day. You will save a lot more which is another reason to minimize eating out.

- In restaurants, try sharing a meal with a friend. Appetizers, entrees, and dessert are good options to share.

- Avoid all-you-can-eat buffets

- Order a low-calorie appetizer or side dish or have the dressing on the side

- Pick smaller size meal options whenever possible

- Stop eating or drinking once you feel full

- Have a glass of water before your meals

2.3 Your mind and food

Researchers focusing on the relationship between food and the human mind believe many different aspects of life that influence what we eat and how much we eat. These aspects include:

- Cultural influences

- Evolutionary changes

- Social settings

- Family behaviors

- Individual behaviors

- Economic status

- Psychological influences

A lot of us use food as a way of coping when our emotions go through changes from depression, anxiety and even feeling happy or celebratory (which is why we also tend to overeat during occasions). Food's ability to provide short-term mood alleviation usually ends up with regret for eating too much and guilt for eating unhealthy foods. Ultimately, our self-image is the one that suffers from our physical changes, such as weight gain, acne, heart diseases and so on.

What role does psychology play in meal planning?

Psychology is behavioral science that considers how and why people act and do what they do. For people wanting to lose weight or become leaner, psychology studies:

- Behavior — Identifies a person's eating patterns and looking at ways to change eating patterns and behaviors.

- Cognition (thinking) — Therapy is conducted to identify self- defeating thinking patterns that contribute to weight management and eating problems

Are you really hungry?

This is a question a lot of us try to understand to determine whether we are hungry or not but plenty of times, we get this wrong. So let's look at some scenarios. Firstly, pretend that you have a scale between 0 to 10 with 0 being hangry and 10 being glutted. True physical hunger usually builds up gradually and it will cause your stomach to growl. If you do not consume any food when you are experiencing true hunger, your body will nag you to do so. You should eat when you experience true hunger which means on a scale of 0 to 10, it should be between 0 to 4.

Here are other ways to know if your hunger is real:

- You feel the desire to eat gets stronger a little bit at a time

- Your stomach starts growling

- You want something filling and nutritious not just craving to eat something sweet or salty or greasy

- Wait for at least 10 minutes before you eat. If you have a craving, this is not true hunger and the feeling will pass. Drink some water and then wait a few more minutes. If you are still hungry, then the hunger is real.

Part of intuitive eating is to begin by checking in with yourself before you start eating or even before you start thinking about food. You need to ask yourself 'How hungry am I?'. Is it really hunger or are you just feel like snacking? Are you continuing to eat because it tastes so good? Or do you want to load up your plate because you're worried you won't get any later? Because we eat the way we eat, we have lost all our true hunger cues.

The good news is that you can, in fact, get your hunger cues in order, knowing when to eat and when to stop. This will take practice but practice does make perfect. Listening to your body is a big process of intuitive eating.

Before You Eat, Try These 4 Things

The next time you feel the urge to eat, give yourself a pause for a minute and check in with your body's signals. Here's how:

- Begin by giving yourself a quick assessment

- Give yourself a mental checklist to go through and make a note of your food triggers. What are your reasons for turning to food? Are you really hungry or just bored? If you are aware and observant of your food habits, you can then take a powerful step towards becoming a mindful eater who knows when they are truly hungry and when they are not.

- Grab a glass of water.

- In the event you find yourself wanting to eat but you don't feel any tummy rumbling, drink a glass of water first.

Plain water can easily provide satiety without any calories plus it also hydrates your body.

- Keep a food log.

- You can use plenty of apps to help you keep a food log or you can also just make a note of it on your calendar- whichever is easier for you. Jot down your hunger levels and what goes into your mouth after this. Write down how you felt and also what you ate if you want to be extremely detailed. You can start seeing the connections between food and you in even just a mere 3 weeks of logging. This can help you see what might trigger different reactions.

Dig for a deeper connection.

When diets and eating plans don't work, it is time to look a little deeper between your connection with food and how you feel. You may be turning to food at times when you do not feel hungry at all and if this happens quite often in your food log, it is time to change your routine. At times when you feel hungry, switch up what you are doing. From working at your computer, get up and go outside to get some fresh air and see how you feel after that. Or if you woke up feeling hungry, drink a glass of water with some lemon- do you still feel like having that Big Breakfast from McDonald's?

What If You Ate, But You Still Feel Hungry?

So you diligently waited until you experienced true hunger, you ate but you still feel hungry after you finished. What gives?

Should you attempt a second serving? Feeling hungry after you eat a reasonable amount of food can happen and it happens for a few reasons which are:

You ate too quickly.

1. The feeling of satiety happens differently between the brain and the stomach and this is due to the interactions that occur with other parts of the body. It takes about 20 minutes for your brain to register the food in your body and that you've eaten enough so if you eat too quickly, your mind might tell you that you still feel hungry. So give yourself time to recognize that your stomach has had enough.

2. You could be a bit dehydrated.

3. Did you sip any water or fluids during your meal or did you even drink that whole glass of water before eating? Try drinking a glass of water and waiting a few minutes to determine if you are really, truly hungry.

4. The food you ate didn't contain enough protein.

5. Most protein-packed foods can help promote satiety so it is a good step to include them in your meals to feel more satisfied. Foods high in protein have been known to increase fullness rating more so than low-protein based foods.

6. You might actually need to eat more.

7. If you have recently stepped up your workout regimen and you've also waited 20 minutes before eating again, chances are that you are hungry and this just means you may need

to eat more. Other signs could also be that you need more calories in your diet and the cues are that you feel irritable, you have trouble sleeping and you are also low on energy. When you do feel this way, it is recommended that you are either more veggies to your daily servings, more fruit or even snack on nuts and seeds.

CHAPTER 3-
WHAT IS MINDFUL EATING?

Practicing mindful eating is one of the best ways to improve your relationship with food. This technique helps you gain control over your food and eating habits and it also promotes sustainable weight loss, reduces binge eating and overall, you feel much better after eating. In this chapter, we will consider what constitutes mindful eating, what you need to know to get started as well as how it works.

3.1 Is it starving?

Mindful eating is not starving the body. It puts awareness on the menu wherever and whenever we eat. It makes us watchful of what we eat and it also aims to transform our relationship with food by focusing on the why and the how of eating, encouraging more sustainable and holistic points of view. This also means that we have better opportunities to understand how food nourishes our bodies and what it can do to keep us healthy. It also helps us create a deeper appreciation for the work that goes into making a meal, savoring every mouthful and every ingredient.

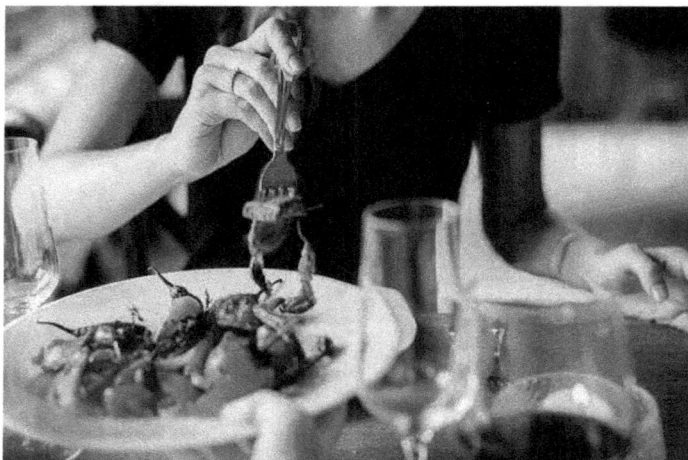

3.2 Is it dieting?

Mindful eating, on its own, is not a diet. It does not have any kind of juice cleanses and neither does it require you to eliminate any kinds of food. It also does not tell you when to eat and there are no promises of quick fixes. Mindful eating is more a framework or guide that helps you eat better and make better choices with your food. It puts you as the decision-maker of all your choices so you choose what to eat to meet your fitness and weight goals. Through mindful eating, you are not eating just as a means to an end, it is not about choosing foods based on our desired outcome. This is potentially self-defeating. All mindful eating does is to invite ourselves to be present while we cook, and eat our foods, to savor without any guilt or judgment, anxiety or inner commentary.

This method is all about spending less time focused on what your weight would be or should be and all kinds of storylines about your weight and instead, embracing eating in a way that

38

helps people find the weight that is right for them. Conventional dieting and eating plans cause too much stress around eating, even if the plan wasn't meant for it to be like that but because we put in heaps of pressure and intensity together with false expectations, most of the time we end up ruining our diet and eating plans.

Through mindful eating, we want to eliminate the view of food being a reward or punishment. Because we view food like this, we end up saying we 'deserve' a huge slice of chocolate cake because we view it as a treat after going through 24 hours of fasting or going one week on a celery juice diet or even eating less than 500 calories for an entire month. People who want to lose weight are obsessed with wanting to be thin that we either end up undereating or suppressing our feelings of hunger or we just end up ignoring our signs of being full.

The issue begins when we internalize ideas built around dieting and we get sucked into the idea that suggests losing weight is as easy as ABC. This is when the emotions and pressures are heightened and we end up sabotaging our diets and plans after a while. Mindful eating is all about encouraging us to let go of the traditional all-or-nothing mindset and refocus our energy on eating according to our natural body weight and not the one shown in magazines or on TV. There is no definite strategy with mindful eating neither is there any calorie-counting on extreme ends. All we are doing is simply trying to be aware.

The mind is calmer when we are more aware and when the mind is calm, we are less agitated or stressed and the less we eat emotionally. When we are more focused, we also increase our clarity to look at the choices we make on food and make better attempts to eat better food choices. When we are calmer and clearer, we are more content, more compassionate on our weight and ourselves and we also become more aware that sustainable weight loss is a journey.

Mindful eating is about bringing mindfulness back to the dining table and this also means a kinder and gentler approach towards eating. It is not about changing our diets but more about changing our relationship and thoughts about food.

3.3 What is mindful eating habits?

As we know, mindful eating is about tuning our bodies and making it more aware of the sensations we experience that precede the 'fullness recognition' in our brains and it also helps us to better gauge our satiation state versus our snacking state even without waiting for 20 minutes. It helps us reach a state of attention on our cravings, our experiences as well as our physical cues.

We reset our ideas of what hunger and full cues are and eliminate cues that we learned as a child such as "You're not leaving the table until you finish your plate!" or "You can't be hungry!" or "Are you sure you need seconds?". Our conditioning with food starts early and we cascade these ideas down to our children to help them listen to their states of hunger and fullness, rather than just ignore them.

Essentially, mindful eating habits include:

- appreciating your food

- eating slowly and without distraction

- Understanding and knowing true hunger and non-hunger triggers for eating

- engaging your senses through colors, smells, sounds, textures, and flavors

- learning to cope with guilt and anxiety about food

- eating to maintain overall health and well-being

- Seeing the effects food has on your feelings and figure

- listening to physical hunger cues and eating only until you're full

These elements allow you to replace automatic thoughts and reactions with more healthier and conscious responses.

3.4 Eating Real Food

Vegetables

No matter what vegetarian diet you are on, vegetables take center stage for all vegetarian diets. However, Vegetables themselves are quite tricky because some of them can be high in carbs whereas some are safe and low in carbs which make excellent choices if you want to decrease your carb intake. So what are low carb vegetables? There is a rule that you can follow.

- Any plants growing ABOVE ground are low in carbs

- Any vegetables growing BELOW ground contain more carbs so either eat them minimally or don't eat them at all.

Essentially, most above-ground vegetables have less than 5 grams of carbs. If you are not on a very strict low-carb diet, you can take in more than 20 grams of carbs per day but if you are on a very strict low carb diet, then never go above 20 grams. Peppers and tomatoes although relatively low in carbs should be taken sparingly as one medium-sized pepper can bring about 6 to 8 grams of carbs.

Beans & Legumes

Corn, beans, lentils, peas, and quinoa are packed with nutrients but aren't very keto-diet friendly. They contain more carbs than vegetables to you might want to be very careful with them. Eat them in small amounts or have none at all.

Grains & Seeds

Let's get one thing clear- wheat isn't a vegetable. It is a grain, and so anything made with wheat flour contains easily digestible carbs so avoid this as much as you can, even if it does say whole grain. Bread, rice, pasta, and all your favorite baked goods are, unfortunately out of the list when it comes to maintaining a keto diet.

Dairy

If you practice a lacto-vegetarian or lacto-ovo vegetarian diet, then great! Butter, cheese, cream, sour cream, Turkish or Greek yogurt become your best friends in the Keto Diet! But just be careful of processed cheese, reduced-fat or skim milk as well as flavored yogurt as they contain loads of sugar and you don't want that. Skip anything that is flavored, low fat, and sugary.

Nuts & Berries

Nuts are full of protein and berries are full of antioxidants, and they are perfect for snacks. However, some nuts are high in carbs and some low. Your best options for nuts are Brazil, macadamia, and pecan nuts. These nuts can be eaten freely even with a strict low-carb diet. These nuts also contain healthy fats making any salad or snacks very satisfying. Walnuts, hazelnuts, pine nuts, peanuts, and almonds contain moderate carbohydrates, but pistachios and cashew nuts are the worst for keto diets. Just two handfuls of cashew bring in a whopping 20 grams!

Beverage

Water, of course, has zero fats, carbohydrates and calories so drink as much water as your body needs. If you are a coffee drinker, then take your coffee entirely black or with full-fat cream. Tea is also excellent on keto-diets. Alcohol? Well, dry red or white wine is fine as with whiskey, brandy, and vodka. Take these clean without sugar. If you like cocktails, eliminate any sugar content.

Candy & Sweets

Stick with dark chocolate, preferably one that has at least 70% cocoa.

Fish & Shellfish

If you are on a pescatarian diet, all kinds of fish get the green light in the Keto diet especially fatty fish such as mackerel, sardines, herring, and salmon. Of course, when eating fish, eat them steamed, grilled, seared or pan-fried. Avoid any breaded fish.

Eggs

Go all out and eat them fried, boiled, scrambled, poached. Eggs are an excellent source of protein and it also helps in packing the protein in keto diets. As with meats, make sure your eggs are also organically sourced and from free-range chickens or ducks.

Sauces & Condiments

Butter and cream are perfectly fine for cooking and making your meals. Not only does it make your food taste better it'll make you more satisfied. But before pouring on that Béarnaise or Hollandaise sauce or ketchup, check your ingredients. You do not want to overload on sugar and artificial ingredients so if you can, make your own sauce or switch to coconut or olive oils for dressing.

AVOID AS MUCH AS YOU CAN:

Sugar

Sugar is your first enemy in a keto-diet. In fact, it's a big culprit for a lot of common diseases such as diabetes and even cancer. So avoid at all costs soft drinks, fruit juices (except cold-pressed), candy, chocolates, cakes and pastries, buns and ice cream, breakfast cereals and sugar-coated anything. Avoid sweeteners as well.

Starch

As mentioned above, any pasta or rice, bread and any forms of potato dishes such as fries, potato chips should be lessened or altogether eliminated. Porridge and muesli are also a no-go. Although whole grain products aren't so bad, best to avoid if possible. Moderate amounts of legumes and root vegetables are found just make sure you eat the extremely low carb version. Beer is also made from wheat, and it is easily absorbed by the body, so avoid if you go out for drinks. Opt for wine or hard liquor. Fruits are also full of sugar but treat them like the natural form of candy, so eat occasionally.

KEEP AN EYE OUT FOR THESE:

We all know by now that supermarkets and grocery stores are packed with low-carb options for food but should you be buying them? One of the main movements of the keto-diet is for us to eat wholesome foods. Low-carb products such as chocolate and pasta work poorly against the keto-diet. Not only that, it further prevents weight loss or a healthier body. Usually, these products come full of carbs that you cannot see. To prevent yourself from becoming a victim of this marketing gimmick, here are two simple rules to follow:

Two simple rules to avoid this junk:

- High carb foods are high-carb. Do not eat low carb versions of it unless you made it yourself or you are 100 percent sure of the ingredients in them.

- Avoid products with ingredients 'net carbs'. That's a marketing gimmick.

Mindfully Eat Wholesomely

Mindful Eating promotes and encourages healthy eating. You eat all types of foods. You focus on eating good quality and wholesome foods and eliminate processed food. Primarily, the food you buy shouldn't come with a list of its ingredients. Here is a useful list of low carb vegetables, moderate carb vegetables as well as high carb vegetables.

LOW-carb vegetables (under 5 grams per serving)	MODERATE-carb vegetables (5-15 grams per serving)	HIGHER-carb vegetables (15-25 grams per serving)
Lettuce	Spaghetti squash	Acorn squash
Spinach	Brussels sprouts	Sweet potatoes
Celery	Broccoli	
Bok choy	Carrots	
Cucumber	Beets	
Radishes	Onion	
Green peppers		
Zucchini		
Cauliflower		
Tomatoes		
Swiss chard		
Kale		
Asparagus		
Turnips		
Mushrooms		

Bottom Line

Once we are able to trace our emotions and also our responses around food and the dynamics at play, we are more equipped to place better decisions to maintain a healthy weight. Food is not a means to an end. It is a source of nutrition to keep our body healthy. We do not need to eat with our feelings but when we do, we learn not to beat ourselves up for it. Eat without having an inner dialogue because you made the right decision to eat and you've eaten the right foods. Look forward to a more carefree, balanced attitude towards food, freed from the shackles of poor eating habits. Step away from unhealthy thoughts about food and cultivate a more sustainable outlook.

We need to re-educate ourselves with food and we need to learn to enjoy our food without guilt or pressure and to eat to live healthily.

CHAPTER 4-

THE EATING BRAIN

Overeating is not a simple issue and this is different for each person. Kim Pearson, nutritionist, and weight loss expert says that to define overeating, to put it simply, it is the excess consumption of food. In this chapter, we will consider ways to reset the thinking process between our stomachs and our brains, create a personal commitment to change as well as creating food rules to follow.

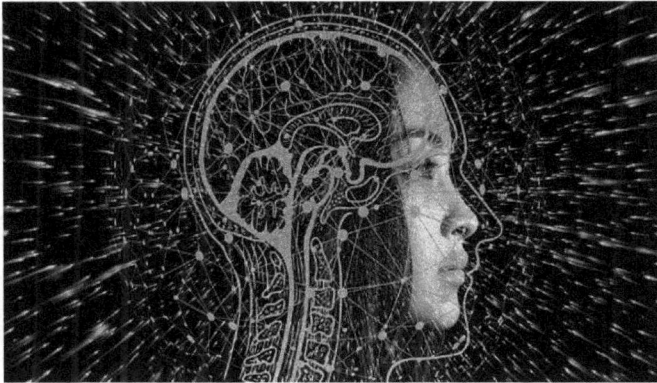

4.1 Resetting

Getting Enough Sleep- One of the best ways Pearson says to curb overeating is simply by getting enough sleep because lack of sleep interferes with the hormones that govern our eating behaviors. When we do not have enough sleep, our levels of hunger hormones which is called ghrelin increases and you are more likely to feel hungrier than usual, which usually leads to overeating. Sleep also regulates the hormone leptin which is the satiety hormone. This hormone lets us know when we have had enough to eat and sends signals to the brain that we are full. Not sleeping enough sleep reduces the levels of leptin and the fullness messages do not get through.

Make at least One Clear Food rule- We did say at some points in this book that eating plans rarely work but there is an exception to that notion. Having a food rule helps you reset your mind and one of those ways is through intermittent fasting. Most people do a 16:8 rule which is fast for 16 hours and your eating window is for 8 hours. Out of those 16 hours, you spend at least 7 to 8 hours sleeping so really, you're fasting for a good 8 hours awake. Other food rules that you can make is that you will only have 1 huge meal a day, it can also be only Saturdays you can eat while watching TV, it can also be no drink 2 liters of water every morning and nothing else, or it could even chew your food slowly with every bite. Whatever rules you put in for yourself it fine so long as you do not restrict yourself from eating enough calories and nutrition.

You can also change your food rules depending on your needs but don't simply change it to make things easier for you to overeat. You want rules that help you reach your goal and objective of a healthier you and a better relationship with food. Allow for at least 7 to 14 days of going through your food rules before changing them, because this way, you've at least given some time to the rule to see if it works for you or not and you aren't just giving up on it. When you have a rule that works for you, your lifestyle and your needs, write it down and set it in stone. You want to be able to see it all the time so that it is ingrained in your mind and you remember it each time you eat or when you wake up.

Separate your constructive and destructive thoughts - This part involves disassociating yourself from destructive and impulsive thoughts about food. You can all these thoughts you Food Monster or Food Demon. Associate a voice or a sound to this demon so that every time you get close to breaking your food rule, this voice or sound is the one you hear. You can also give it a name, such as Evil Butter or Demon Dana. This idea is to help you recognize and ignore that inner voice that has been responsible for all your bad choices around food.

For example, your food rule could be 'No drinking coffee for more than twice a day'. But you end up passing by a Starbucks and you think 'You deserve another cup of coffee after all the work you put in today' or you could also think 'Nope, it's full of caffeine and it's bad for you'. If you have these thoughts, you can instead say to yourself 'I do not want coffee, my Food Demon wants it and it wants Evil Butter! I never eat Evil Butter!"

As crazy as this sounds, it is a primitive technique to help you decide in those microseconds of moments to remember who you are and why you made those rules in the first place. This is not a miracle mantra but it does help you restore your sense of power and association with food, especially if you've been struggling to overcome your bad food habits for a long time.

4.2 Self-discipline and creating a Commitment to Change

Our food demon will not be controlled unless we have the discipline to know why we have these rules and establish them. So when creating your food rules, here are a few things to think about:

1. What are the things that are most important to you in life?

2. What are the things that you want to do in this life?

3. What are your values and beliefs when it comes to food?

4. What are your health and fitness goals?

5. What weight do you feel you can be happy with and which is healthy for you?

When doing this exercise, remember that creating your mission statement isn't a one-time thing that's set in stone. Give yourself the opportunity to review your mission statement focused on your health annually and see if it has resulted in aligning positively with your life, career, jobs, and relationships. Adjust if necessary.

One of the first few things anyone must do to become self-disciplined is to make a personal commitment. Your commitment should be that from this day forward, you are going to do the things you know you must do, abide by the food rules you make and when must you do them. This commitment must include the rule that you cannot allow yourself to make excuses or justify why you aren't doing what you are supposed to be doing.

Yes, it's hard to do but the key here is to start small. Doing small changes in your daily life will help you towards becoming self-disciplined. Start your day by waking up early. If your regular wake up time is at 8 am, then make it 7.30 am. Make your bed or empty the trash. Drink a glass of water. Do 10-minutes of stretching or meditation. All these tiny things are what get you en route to become more disciplined. Robert Collier wisely said 'Success if the sum of small efforts, repeated day in day out'. Becoming disciplined may seem like the hardest thing you can do, but the rewards are immense. A successful life is built on a foundation of discipline.

Building Your Commitment to Change

Commitment is all about being dedicated to doing something, to act to bring out the desired result. It is the dedication to take action. Make no mistake that commitment is a result of an external force. No- commitment is an internally motivated feature. You need to be willing to take action because you care about the results. For successful and sustainable change, you need this level of commitment. This is what fuels a person's desire to take the next step, to keep things on going and to always look for solutions whenever there's a problem. So how do you know the strength of commitment that you have for your professional or personal goals?

Firstly, all of us have commitments that are about things and issues that we care about. For instance, you may be displaced by the discomfort you feel right now about how things are, or you may feel the yearning for something better. You may also be moved by an exciting challenge to create something new for yourself or your company. So, ask yourself- what is it that is important to me and why do I need to change? What are the things I care most about? The change will never be achieved without any commitment. We need to have a strong commitment that engages us to change and to sustain.

Act to Build Commitment for Change

Follow these guidelines to help you make a strong commitment to change:

- Express and Demonstrate Change - Always remember that change does not come from a large organization, rather it's the people that change. You need to express and demonstrate your commitment to your health goals to influence change. An environment of change needs to be created to encourage others to commit. When the people around you see this commitment, they will continue supporting you.

- Be clear on your purpose to change- To make a change is to have a clear focus. If your health agenda is clear with measurable results, you will not lose sight of your goals.

- Invite Reflection- Reflecting on what you have done and how you have worked before to attain your previous goals will help you achieve your future ones. Sometimes looking back helps you pinpoint what exactly went wrong or how best to improve on this.

- Make room for emotional change- Allow yourself to express discomfort, excitement, fear or sadness. You are after all human and making changes is a big thing in anyone's lives. So, you will be experiencing different emotions along the path to glory. Adjust along the way if you need to.

- Be free to commit- Don't restrict yourself when it comes to changing. Just understand that change takes time and energy, so don't expect to launch in a series of different changes at one go and expect yourself to commit immediately.

- Follow Through- When you have committed yourself to change, you need to make sure that you clearly demonstrate the actions that are required to make that change. Start small and keep the momentum going till you reach your personal best, and then it's time to reinvent and make new changes- keep the wheel going. Never stop re-inventing.

4.3 No hunger rule- Hara Hachi Bu

Have you heard of Hara Hachi Bu? This is a Japanese practice that is about eating until you are 80 percent full. A lot of us grew up with the notion that we need to finish the food on our plates otherwise you do not leave the dining table. As a child, you needed to finish your food to get dessert. This style of eating did not consider how full you are, how you would feel if you took another bite and what amount of food your body needed. It also prevented us from listening to our body's needs. By practicing Hara Hachi bu, you eat only until you are 80 percent full and this helps us all learn to eat at a certain ratio rather than counting calories and being stressed all throughout. While we all do not know what 80 percent full actually feels like, we do know that if we eat until we are full, we are most likely to feel full after 20 minutes because that is how long the stomach takes to communicate with the brain that it is full. This brings us to our next question- what is 80 percent full for the human body?

According to Susan Dopart, a registered dietician, it takes about 15 to 20 meals to reset the muscle memory of the stomach for it to get used to the less food idea and we need to allow and trust for this process to happen. We are all used to eating until we are full and this is always past our satiety rate which is why it is hard for us to lose weight. So, the best way, according to Susan Dopart is to eat just half of what you would normally eat and to check to see if you are full. When we begin to feel any stomach pressure, this is when Ms. Dopart says we are at 80% full stage. From here on, if you continue eating, you are eating not because you are hungry, you are only eating until you are full. Remember that you need to go through a process of at least 20 meals before your brain registers this feeling and from then on, you continue eating until you are 80% full and never more. Your biggest challenge is to learn to listen to your body, being aware of the signs and to honor them.

That's it for now. Good luck.

CHAPTER 5-
SCIENCE OF WEIGHT LOSS

5.1 Should I start dieting?

It is a very subjective thing and there is no immediate yes or immediate no because there are many ways to diet. There are healthy ways that produce sustainable results and there are unhealthy ways that might lead to having an eating disorder and there are also crash diets that enable you to lose pounds quickly but is not very sustainable.

Whatever your reasons are, before you begin to diet, you need to determine why you want to diet:

- Is it just to lose weight?

- Are you going into surgery?

- Are you trying to cut back on certain food items like carbs and sugar?

- Are you pre-diabetic?

- Do you have some other health issues?

- Are you planning to include exercise?

For successful weight loss and sustainable weight management, a positive attitude is important and you also need to make a commitment to adopt healthier habits and healthier ways of life.

The good news is that you can control your weight (unless there is a medical issue) and usually, to lose weight you need to reduce your calorie intake or burn up more calories than you consume. For sustainable and healthy weight loss, you need to do both. Oftentimes when people follow or begin a low-calorie diet, they can feel deprived and it can increase the temptation to binge and it also reduces your muscle and not fat. Instead of looking fit and toned, you have a body that jiggles which is why incorporating bodyweight exercises helps to tone and tighten.

To answer the question of whether you should start dieting- ask yourself those questions above and think about what you want in terms of health and fitness. Dieting may be useful if you are cutting down on calories gradually and opting for healthier choices of food.

Remember that dieting alone is not the key to sustainable weight loss. Research has shown that people who follow diets (extremely) usually gain their weight back once they stop. Your best solution is to switch your eating habits, incorporate healthier choices, lean meats, and wholesome foods and exercise for at least 30 minutes every day.

How many calories do I need?

For people who plan on starting a diet, the immediate element they consider is calories. While cutting calories help, it is not the be everything, end all because everyone's energy needs are different and in order to function in optimal capacity and prevent malnutrition, you need to look into your daily needs, your body composition, height, weight as well as fitness.

That said, there are ways to estimate how many calories you require in a day. A quick and simple way is to look at your daily activity level- how active or sedentary are you. Here are some definitions you can consider:

- **Low activity**- you rarely workout or exercise or you are only involved in physical activities during the weekends.

- **Moderate:** your workout or exercise at least three times a week for 30 minutes a day

- **High:** your workout and exercise at least 4 to 6 times a week for a minimum of 30 minutes to 60 minutes a day.

Next, find your activity factor by using the chart below. Look for the number where your activity level matches your weight status. Multiply this activity factor by your weight to estimate how many calories are needed to maintain your current weight.

To lose weight: Subtract 250 calories to lose 1/2 pound per week. Subtract 500 calories to lose 1 pound per week.

Underweight

Underweight

Low activity: 16

Moderate activity: 18

High activity: 22

Normal Weight

Low activity: 14

Moderate activity: 16

High activity: 18

Overweight

Low activity: 11

Moderate activity: 14

High activity: 16

- Making every calorie count

If you are looking for a tool to help you meet your nutritional needs while losing weight, check out the USDA's MyPlate resource. It gives you good guidance on eating balanced and proper meals to help you not only lose weight but also improve your nutrition. Check it out here: www.choosemyplate.gov.

- Keeping track

As mentioned before, keeping a food journal or an app can help you track your food and eating habits. Be as detailed as possible from your moods to the type of day, the weather and how your eating habits are like these days. Include your serving sizes as well as what you drink. Be accurate and be honest- this will be helpful for you to see what needs to be changed, what needs to be kept and what can be improved in terms of eating habits, behaviors as well as food choices.

- Putting it all together

Mildly restricting calories or eliminating a food group from your daily nutritional intake, changing your diet as well as keeping track of what you consume will only be sustainable if exercise is incorporated into your schedule. This will make your weight loss efforts sustainable and healthy.

5.2 Should I start intermittent eating?

That depends- what are your body or weight goals? According to Carly Pollack, a Certified Clinical Nutritionist as well as a Lifestyle Coach at Nutritional Wisdom, says that our body is designed to burn energy by using glucose or fat. When you make your body become adapted to fat as fuel, it will start using fat for energy instead of carbohydrates broken into glucose.

When you intermittent fast, you create a superior environment for your body to burn fat. Of course, there are other benefits to intermittent fasting which we will consider in this book. This involves cancer prevention, longevity, improved digestion as well as insulin resistance. So, the bottom line is, doing intermittent fasting is a personal choice based on what your health goals are. You can go on an intermittent fast to kick start a more superior process of your digestive system, lose weight healthily and reap the benefits of having better insulin tolerance.

Who should not try intermittent fasting?

Just like other diets and eating plants, intermittent fasting is also not for everyone. There are medical conditions that prevent people from taking on intermittent fasting.

The main issues are:

- People with a history of eating disorders

- People who are currently underweight.

- People are recovering from illness or injury.

- People who have Type 1 diabetes mellitus.

- People with low blood pressure (hypotension).

- Women who are trying to conceive

- Women who are pregnant

The reason why those in the group above are listed is that while there are positive benefits, there could be risks of impairment, risk of dangerously low sugar levels or even the risk of not getting enough nutrition. Now that you have an idea of who can and who cannot go on intermittent fasting, let's have a look at a few basic things regarding this fast.

Women, especially women who are suffering from hormonal imbalances, adrenal dysfunction, any other sort of bodily imbalance and even those who suffer from thyroid problems should be very wary about starting an intermittent fasting plan. You can consult your doctor beforehand and just consult with them if this is going to be a safe bet for you or not, but if you are thinking about starting this eating regime, you should be cautious as it may cause your body more harm than good.

Women with PCOS, for example, could experience problems with intermittent fasting because it will begin to take its toll on your body and regular fasting may be in danger of causing your body more stress instead of helping it get healthier. Among some of the problems that women with hormonal imbalances could encounter if they undergo the intermittent fasting program includes acne, depression, stress, and even disruptions in your menstrual cycle.

The bottom line is that women with any kind of hormonal imbalances should not be doing intermittent fasting because your body is already not functioning the way that a healthy body should, and fasting is only going to increase the severity of the imbalances you are already experiencing. Intermittent fasting is great, that is unless you have adrenal, thyroid or autoimmune issues. Although intermittent fasting is supposed to be the way to get your health back on track again, it isn't going to work as well for those who are already not in the peak of health because you're most likely already struggling. Pregnant women should stay well away from intermittent fasting too because you are at a stage where your body needs to have all the nutrients it can get to feed the growing baby inside of you. Weight gain is to be expected during pregnancy, that is just something that you have to deal with, it's a packaged deal.

Understanding How Intermittent Fasting Works

To understand how intermittent fasting will benefit us, we need to first understand how our bodies work, and this applies to both men and women. At its core, our body functions primarily in two states – it is either fed, or it is fasting (when it's not being given food).

When our body is in a fed state, it is working to digest and absorb the calories from the food we eat. Generally, we are in a fed state during our waking others, because of the need that fuel and that energy to get through a busy day from morning to night when we can go to bed again.

When we go to bed is when we are in a fasted state, because for a good 8 hours at the very least, our bodies have no access to food or calories. When our bodies have no access to extra calories, it then turns its focus to burning the excess fat which is stored in our bodies. This is what the foundation of intermittent fasting is based upon.

It requires you intentionally putting your body through a certain time frame where it isn't being given any calories through food during your waking hours. This will allow your body to go into its fat-burning mode, using the fat in our bodies as energy for you to get through the day until your next meal.

This simply means that instead of eating three meals a day of breakfast, lunch, and dinner, you are now only going to be eating two meals. Which meal you skip is dependent upon your preference. What happens when you eat one less meal a day? You're already consuming fewer calories than you normally would, and fewer calorie intake is how your body begins to lose the extra pounds.

When we eat, not all the calories and energy from food is going to be used immediately. Our bodies will take what we need,

64

and store the rest away for later. There's one key hormone that is involved in storing this energy, and that hormone is called insulin.

Whenever we eat, the insulin in our body rises, which then helps to store the excess energy which is either stored in our liver or stored in other fat deposits in our bodies. When we fast, the process gets reversed. Insulin levels begin to drop, which then gives our bodies the cue that it is time to start digging into that stored away energy, and that's when the body begins breaking down the fat and using it as energy.

5.3 Count for calories

Calories, calories, calories. Do you know what they are? Essentially, calories are just a way to measure energy and it is usually a system used to measure energy content in the foods we eat and the things we drink. A dietary calorie, technically speaking is defined as the amount of energy that is needed to raise the temperature of 1 kg of water by 1 degree Celsius. These calories from food and drink are important for essential functions such as thinking and breathing, walking to running, studying, focusing and pretty much all our day-to-day activities. All other calories not used will be stored as fats. Eating more than you burn will also account for stored calories which in turn makes you put on weight.

Why Calories Count?

Plenty of articles and journals and even doctors will tell you that calories do not matter and that it is a waste of time. But there are also doctors and nutritionists, journals and magazines that will tell you that calorie counting is important. It depends on who you speak with and what reasons do you talk about calories. When it comes to weight though, calories are a deciding factor. It helps to know what your calorie intake should be for your body type and it also helps you set goals that are healthy. It also helps to know what is considered a low-calorie diet and what a balanced calorie diet would look like.

It has been proven in scientific experiments called overfeeding studies time and time again where subjects are asked to deliberately overeat and then the impact on their weight and health is measured. Research has found that when you consume more calories than you burn, you will gain weight. So, in trying to intuitively and mindfully eat, keeping in mind the calories you consume will help you create an eating plan that is both nutritious and enough to prevent you from overeating.

Tips to Succeed with Calorie Counting

Here are 5 more tips to count calories:

Before we go into the tips, keep in mind that you DO NOT WANT TO BE OBSESSED with calorie counting. A few calories outside the determined intake will not wreak havoc on your system so long as it does not happen frequently. Calorie counting is merely a guide.

- Be prepared: Before you start, download a calorie counting app or online tool, to help you measure or estimate your portions and make a **meal plan**.

- Read food labels: These labels contain loads of information that is useful for counting calories. Make sure you check the portion size recommended on the package.

- Remove temptation: Clean out your fridge and pantry and get rid of snacks, processed foods and sugary items to make it easier to help you stick and hit your calorie targets.

- Aim for slow, steady weight loss: Do not abruptly cut calories. While you may be able to lose weight faster, remember that it will not last. You want to give your body time to adjust to changes. Slow and steady is the way and you are more likely to stick to your plan.

- Fuel your exercise: Any weight loss is successful if it includes exercise. Not only will it make you lose weight faster, but it will also help you tone your body and increase your energy. Just make sure that you continue eating well to supplement the energy that goes into your exercises

Bottom Line

While knowing the calorie intake your body needs is helpful, it is not the be-all, end-all. It is not the only thing that is required for optimal health. Counting calories helps you stay on your target and understand food and nutrition better. It also helps you make better food choices. It may not suit everyone, but you may find that counting calories are an effective way to lose weight and keep it off.

CHAPTER 6-
MINDFUL MEAL PREPPING
FOR WEIGHT LOSS

Essentially, meal prep is many things to different people because of the different fitness goals or different routines and personal requirements. Meal prep is a short form for meal preparation and what entails is a process of planning, preparing and packaging meals in advance usually covering the entire week or upcoming weeks. The primary reason for meal prepping is for clean eating and portion control. But as mentioned, it is a different reason for everyone although ultimately, it does lead to eating a balanced meal, having fewer additives and artificial flavoring in your meals because you know what you put into your cooking.

Some people choose to only meal prep breakfasts or lunches whereas some meal prep dinners or maybe all the meals, which includes snacks. Whatever the reason or whatever way they choose to do it, meal prep involves experimenting with what works right for you until you find a routine that works seamlessly with your schedule.

Meal prepping allows you to plan your meals, go grocery shopping, cook your meals and pack them. Ideally, you get to pick and choose what kind of foods you eat, what goes into your food and how big or small those portions are. Depending on what your fitness goals are, you can make a low-carb meal, high-protein meals, a balanced meal and so many more.

6.1 Benefits of Meal Prepping

Here are some benefits of meal preparation:

- **You will save money**

If you thought eating healthily is expensive, here is some news for you- it doesn't have to be if you plan. Buying in bulk helps reduce prices significantly. Also, meal prepping requires heavy use of the freezer. Planning your meals in advance enables you to know exactly how much you need to buy, where to buy them and stock on ingredients.

- You will lose weight

Knowing what goes into your body and how much will ultimately lead to gradual and healthy weight loss. You don't need to diet; you don't need to cut down. You just need to focus on healthy and wholesome additions to your meal which means no processed foods, no sugary stuff and so on. Prepping on a weekly basis also allows you to control your calories.

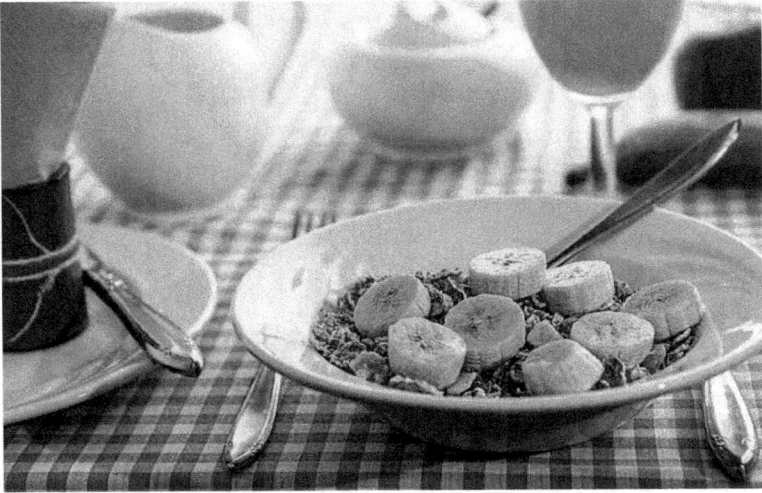

- Grocery shopping will not be a headache

If grocery shopping is a nightmare to you all these while, it is only because you don't know what to buy when you walk into the store and see rows and rows of food items. Once you know what you are going to cook for the whole week, your aimless wondering will be reduced and so will the time spent in the grocery store. With your list, you can head to the aisles to get your fruits, veggies, dairy, grains, and protein. Being focused also reduces the chances of wondering about the processed food section.

- You will learn how to portion control

Meal preparation teaches you the art of balance. The whole idea of meal prepping is to prepare your meals and pack them into containers and by doing so, it makes you inclined to only put in a certain amount of food into the food containers. Also, it prevents you from eating more so that stops you from overeating too. Part of losing weight is consuming the right amount of food for your physical needs. You are still able to treat yourself but even that can be meal prepped. The basic idea is that you can ensure you get your recommended nutrients and you also monitor the amount of food you eat.

- Your food wastage also reduces

Meal preparation also reduces food wastage because you end up utilizing all your ingredients for the week when you meal prep at the beginning of each week. It is also very unlikely that you'll have any leftover at the end of the week.

- You will also save time

You only need to invest a certain amount of time at the beginning of the week to plan, prep, cook, and pack. After that, you save time away from the kitchen and the only time you need to spend time in the kitchen is to heat up your food. You don't need to figure out what to cook every day, and make a last-minute and frequent trips to the store each time you want to cook something.

- You will be investing in your health

Meal prepping allows you plan on what you'll be eating throughout the week. People who meal prep have a high chance of eating cleaner and healthier than those who do not. You also will be more focused on your meals and wouldn't be finding something to eat and risk eating something unhealthy. Good nutrition contributes to better overall health.

- You will have better willpower

Meal prepping gets you into a routine and over time, you'd find yourself eating healthily more consistently. The more you meal prep breakfast, lunch, dinner, and snacks, the more you'll realize that you have less and less cravings and prevent binge eating.

- It will reduce stress

Walking about aimlessly in a grocery store is a cause for stress. Not knowing what to eat daily is also a cause for stress. Stress can affect your mind and body in various easy. It can have an adverse effect on your digestive system for starters which will then lead to disruptive sleeping patterns and affect your immune system. Meal prepping will stop you from saying 'What's for lunch or What's for Dinner'. Instead, you'll probably reach out to whatever packed food in your fridge, heat it and eat it. It makes more time for yourself and family, you have more time to relax, especially on weekdays and you will have good food to eat.

- You will have a variety of things to eat

As mentioned before, meal prepping requires some form of experimentation. More often than not, you'll also learn from trial and error. But eventually, you will learn what works for you and what doesn't. You will learn how to use ingredients and food better, how long they last, how to store them and so on. In the process of meal planning, you will also become better at choosing what kind of foods work well as a combination of grains, protein, vegetables and so on. Meal prepping is all about variety so mix and match to ensure a balanced meal.

There are all some of the main benefits of meal prepping. Of course, plenty of people will have other benefits to this. No matter what, always experiment with your meal preps and use the freshest ingredients available to you and the climate that you live in. In the next few chapters, we will explore the psychology of eating and meal prepping, the essentials that you need and many other components of meal prepping.

6.2 Psychology of Meal Prepping

Meal prepping teaches us, over time, to make healthier and mindful decisions with our food choices, thus improving our relationship with food. Meal prepping also teaches us to control our compulsive eating and binging- it enables us to take charge of our appetite. By picking and choosing your food ingredients in the market, coming home and cutting, peeling, chopping and dicing and then moving on to sautéing, cooking, roasting, steaming and so on- you have put in plenty of effort into making your food.

These steps have made you take charge of your appetite through food preparation. While it may seem like a daunting task at first and granted, there could have been plenty of times that things have gone wrong, you ultimately made a meal. Taking charge and cooking something edible makes a person feel calm and increase the alertness to the foods that you eat. Meal prepping changes plenty of deep-seated and unhealthy relationships with food and promotes, among others:

- Better body movement

- Positive body image

- Positive relationships with food

- Increased alertness and energy levels

- Makes eating healthy not so challenging

6.3 Meal Prepping and Weight Management

Meal prepping and weight management look at:

A person's readiness to change- meal prepping takes effort and this includes a high level of awareness of what is required to be done to achieve a week of meals. It takes commitment to plan, shop, cook, and store.

Learning to self-monitor- Meal prepping makes you more aware of the triggers that make you want to munch on something in the moment. It makes you more mindful of your food choices as well as the portions. It tells you what portions make you satiated. It also helps you stay focused on your long-term health goals.

Making alternatives- meal prepping teaches us to minimize distraction by replacing unhealthy food items with healthier alternatives at home and work.

Practicing Psychological Meal Prepping Behaviors

- **Don't** skip meals.
- **Do** keep track of your eating habits
- **Do** limit night eating.
- **Do** drink plenty of water.
- **Do** distract yourself from thinking about food
- **Do** focus on other activities
- **Do** exercise instead of eating when you are bored.

- **Do** watch your portion sizes.

- **Do allow yourself to eat a range of food** without restricting yourself a particular food.

- **Do** give yourself encouragement.

- **Do** think of eating as a lifestyle change.

- **Do use the scale mindfully**. Weigh yourself no more than once a week.

- **Do** make healthy food choices.

By getting ourselves involved with meal preparation, we pay more attention to our food and savor the food we eat much better than purchasing it off a rack or buying it in the store or eating at a restaurant. Most of these ways of eating are momentary and last as long as we eat it but it fades off once we are full and satiated.

Meal prepping allows us to be more grateful, mindful and appreciating of what goes into our mouths and the source of where it came from.

CHAPTER 7-

DRINK AWAY THE EXCESS WEIGHT

Have you heard about how water is an effective element of effective weight loss? In this chapter, we are going to focus on water, specifically water fasting.

In previous chapters, we discussed how drinking water before a meal or starting the day by drinking at least 2 liters of water helps curb cravings as well as increase the feeling of satiety. In this chapter, however, we focus on water fasting and how it can help with losing excess weight.

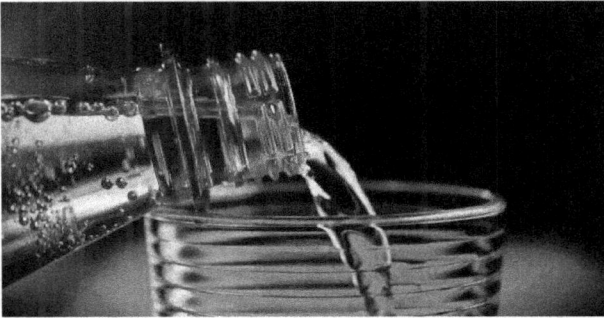

7.1 What Is Water Fasting?

Essentially, water fasting is just another type of fast that only allows you to consume water. These fasts usually can be between 24 hours to 72 hours. During this time, a person does not consume any kind of food and only consumes water.

It is strongly advised not to fast any longer than the period of 24 to 72 hours unless you have medical clearance and under supervision. Why would anyone want to fast for that long? There are plenty of reasons why a person would go fasting by only consuming water. These reasons are:

- For religious purposes

- For spiritual reasons

- To detox the body of toxins

- For the health benefits of fasting

- To prepare for a medical procedure or operation

Plenty of people undertake a water fast for its health benefits and it is also because there are plenty of benefits related to a water fast such as lowering the risk of cancer, diabetes as well as heart diseases.

Water fasting has been known to promote a process called **autophagy** where the body can break down and recycle parts of the cells that may be dangerous. Diets such as the lemon detox have been fashioned after the water fast. The lemon detox fast allows you to drink, several times a day, a mixture of water, lemon juice with a little bit of cayenne pepper or maple syrup added into it for up to seven days. Where water fasting is concerned, while it does have its health benefits, it is not without its risks and it can be dangerous if the fast is prolonged.

What happens in the 24 to 72 hours of a water fast?

During a water fast, you can only drink water and not consume any kind of food or even beverage such as juices.

During a water fast, you need to drink at least two to three liters of water each day, between 24 to 72 hours. Never, ever go beyond this point of time to fast without medical supervision. Confining yourself to an all-water diet for more than 72 hours is hazardous to your health, doing more harm than good.

While in a water fast, it is easy to feel dizzy or weak, especially if you are new to this. During this time, low-intensity work is best so avoid operating heavy machinery, rigorous exercise or even high-intensity workouts.

What happens to your body when you fast?

The first few hours into the fast are pretty normal. People usually can last without feeling dizzy or weak. This is because your body is going through its regular process of storing glucose and breaking down glycogen. In most circumstances, 25% of glucose goes directly to the brain whereas the rest is used to support your muscles and blood cells.

After about five to six hours, most people reach a state of ketosis. This depends on your body's sugar levels- some people take faster and some people take a slower time to reach ketosis. Ketosis is the metabolic state of the body, where energy levels are supported by ketones in your blood. This is the process of breaking down fat. This is when the real fasting begins and it is the most desirable state to be in for people fasting to lose weight. This state can also be reached through a ketogenic diet which is a low-carb, high-fat diet.

When your body goes into ketosis, other things tend to happen such as the release of cholesterol as well as uric acid into the bloodstream. This is an essential process because it detoxifies the body.

At this stage, most people start experiencing dizziness, headaches, skin rashes even as well as fatigue. The lesser-known symptoms are that of muscle pain and joint aches. At the ending of this stage, the pain begins to lessen and the blood pressure will drop. This process is called the calcification process where the mucoid plaque, as well as the cholesterol in the body, will reduce.

When our food intake has been reduced, this gives our digestive system a rest. However, since the process of digestion takes a little time, it is never fully stopped when we fast intermittently. The digestive process fully rests only when we go through a more prolonged fast.

After the first 6 hours of fasting, you will end up feeling hungry, naturally and slightly overwhelmed. This could trigger certain emotional states such as frustration, anger, sadness and even feeling down.

If you are fasting for an extended period, allow yourself to deal with these emotions as they come and to keep telling yourself that the way you feel is happening due to the fast you are undergoing. You do not want to take out your emotions on the people around you which is why fasting also should come with meditation. This helps because it takes your mind away from the hunger and instead focuses it on activities that you can do without much bodily effort.

7.2 The Stages of Water Fasting

Stage 1

The first stage usually starts from the time you take your last meal and lasts up to

about 12-48 hours. Before embarking on this type of fast, it is always recommended that proper planning way ahead to ensure the successful completion of the fasting period.

The first stage is typically the most challenging stage that you would have to go through at the beginning of the fast. At this stage, you will begin to feel hunger pangs due to your normal meal cycles as your body start to adjust itself during this fasting phase. It is also not uncommon to feel low in energy or end up in negative mood swings during this period.

The feeling of 'low energy" occurs when the body starts to adapt during this fasting period when it starts to use less energy. This includes lowering your blood pressure and as well as your heart rate. This process is called "gluconeogenesis", and it is a process where the liver starts to convert fats and amino acids into glucose to obtain the energy it needs for proper bodily functions.

Stage 2

Stage two begins after the first forty-eight hours and will last right up to the seventh day. At this phase, changes in your physical appearance will start to occur and you are entering what is known as "ketosis". At this stage, the body will start to convert the fat stored in your body as fuel. Hence, you might stop feeling moody and hungry during this period.

Stage 3

Stage three will take place from days eight to fifteen and you will start to experience changes to your mood. At this stage, your body becomes fully adjusted to the "fasting" stage and your digestive system goes into a "relaxation" phase. Since you haven't been consuming any solid food or liquids for the better part of the last ten days, the body and digestive system have less work to do in breaking down foods into the bloodstream. When you have entered this phase, you will notice an improvement to your overall wellbeing and increased energy levels plus an improved clarity of mind.

Stage 4

Day sixteen and beyond is when you have entered stage four of the fasting experience. This will then continue towards the end of the fasting period. We advise that if you do reach this stage, you should consult your doctor and ensure the continuation of this stage is done under your doctor's supervision. Stage four of the fasting process is the culmination of the repairing and cleansing process of your body that began with the earlier stages. As such, the longer you fast, the more time the body has the chance to heal itself.

Stage 5

When to break a fast is subjective and it depends totally up to you and your goals. It is important that when you choose to break your fast, you should take your time to re-adjust to consuming solid foods. Your body and digestive system needs time to re-configure back into its normal routine after such a long period of an extended fast. It's best that you ease your way back into this by consuming soups and vegetables as a start. Also, consuming fruit juices will also help accomplish the fast-breaking phase.

7.3 How to prepare your body

Planning is a key component in the successful completion of the water fast. Therefore, it is imperative that you should begin preparing your body and mind in the best way possible during this period. First and foremost, it is ultimately important to seek medical consultation from your doctor before getting into this type of fast. Should you not be in the best shape, the risks that can occur will far outweigh the benefits that can be derived from fasting. Also, those experiencing any medical conditions such as low blood pressure, diabetes, those who are underweight and women in pregnancy should avoid fasting. As such, a proper medical examination to clear yourself as fit before undertaking this type of fast is critical.

The fasting period will cause a lot of changes to your mental state as well. Since you will be experiencing bouts of hunger during the initial stages of the fast, it is also important to prepare mentally for the challenge ahead. So, it is important to ease yourself during the initial stages by being aware and controlling your hunger pangs and mood swings that can occur due to low energy levels. You may also be affected by diarrhea, headaches, fatigue and body odor due to the elimination of waste and toxins in your body. To accommodate these effects, you could opt to take some time off work to put yourself in a relaxed environment and ease your way into the entire fasting process.

You should start this process slowly by "detoxifying" your body. Begin by eliminating foods such as meats, eggs, fish, milk, and cheese. Stop drinking coffee, sugary drinks, and even alcohol. If you are a smoker, best to gradually reduce your smoking habits and coming to a complete stop just before your fasting period is scheduled to begin. Alter your eating habits by consuming more raw and wholesome foods such as vegetables, fruits and grains. And slowly start to consume less and less food as you head towards your fasting deadline.

You may also prepare your body a few weeks ahead before your water fast by utilizing the intermittent fasting method to get your body prepared and train yourself to control your hunger pangs. A simple four-week plan would be as follows:

1. Week 1: Skip eating breakfast

2. Week 2: Skip both breakfast and lunch

3. Week 3: Skip all three meals and control your portions for dinner

4. Week 4: Water Fast begins!!!

In the week or days leading up to the start of your fast, you will need to increase your water intake to prepare your body for the fast period and to ensure it is well hydrated. Lastly, ensure that you get enough sleep and rest before and during your fasting period to ensure your body is fully rested and recovered pre and during your fasting window.

7.4 Weight Loss Benefits of Water Fasting

Now, the big question that those who are keen on losing weight will be curious to know - *does water fasting help with weight loss?*

It will, but there is a difference between losing weight and *burning fat*. Water fasting is not going to help you with the latter. Which means that the majority of your weight loss is going to be a result of your body losing water, muscle mass during the fast and carbs. Not so much about fat burning. In general, it takes several days for the human body to start using their fat stores as fuel, so if you're after a fast fat burning fasting method, another approach may suit you better.

Of course, that's not to say that no weight loss is going to happen. There will be some amount of weight loss benefits that you'll experience with the water fast, especially if you do it consistently. Everyone's bodies work differently; some experience a greater level of weight loss than others. With the water fast method, the first initial stages are going to involve a loss in water weight, and the fat burning only kicks it at a later stage when your body has been deprived of food long enough.

Toronto-based acupuncturist and chiropractor, Ben Kim, mentions that at least one pound a day of weight loss can be expected when undergoing the water fast (again, not everyone's bodies are going to work the same way). Some people may even lose as much as 3 pounds a day, especially if you've previously consumed a diet that involves a large number of processed foods where a lot of water has been retained. Whether we like it or not, there is no one, sure-fire approach method to weight loss. Water fasting, while highly beneficial for your body, on its own is not enough to encourage long-term weight loss. The Academy of Nutrition and Dietetics recommends the best approach to long-term, sustained weight loss as a combination of both healthy diets and exercise.

A Quick Word of Advice

As with any other fasting method, exercise regime or change in your routine, it is always best to consult your doctor or health professional before embarking on a new process. A doctor who is already familiar with your medical history and background would be the best option in this instance because they will be able to advise you about what you need to be cautious of and how to take care of yourself during the fasting period. Talk to your health professional about what your goals are, why you're choosing to undergo this fasting method and about what to expect. At any point when you find yourself feeling unwell, you should stop and consult your health professional immediately.

CHAPTER 8-
FRUITS AND WEIGHT LOSS

sk any health aficionado, vegan or vegetarian or clean eaters about eating fruits and vegetables and they will immediately know what you are referring to. However, when people talk about fruits for weight loss, it always concerns a particular group of food items that claim to have potent vitamins and minerals. This group of food items refers to superfoods!

8.1 The Origins of the Superfood Concept

Type in superfood in Google, click on Images, and you can find a variety of nuts, beans, berries, seeds, roots, and protein that constitute the term superfood. In the developed world, the term superfood is often practiced and said by the public and with a growing interest in the health and food scene. While there is no legal definition of the word superfood, the Oxford dictionary does describe superfoods as "a nutrient-rich food considered to be especially beneficial for health and well-being". The Merriam-Webster dictionary explains superfoods as 'nutrient-dense food, loaded with vitamins, minerals, fiber, antioxidants, and/or phytonutrients". So essentially, Superfoods are food items that have more health benefits or above-average benefits than other foods.

Is there really such a thing as Superfoods?

While there is certainly hype about different food items being extremely nutrient-dense than other food items, it is always a good thing to look at scientific research and evidence. It is a widely known fact that blueberries are well-known as a superfood, and they have been used in regular studies by scientists. Blueberries have a high content of antioxidants; especially the compound chemical called anthocyanins. This chemical compound inhibits and kills the growth of cancerous cells in the human body. Blueberries are a very much sought after superfood in the beauty and wellness section as it is known to slow down and even reverse age-related skin conditions.

Antioxidants have been widely recognized as molecules that protect the cells in the body from harmful UV rays and free radicals that come from everyday exposure to things like smoke and sun, foods and weather and so on. While the body does produce these molecules naturally, the fact that there are too many free radicals in the body can result in oxidative stress, which then causes cell damage. This imbalance of free radicals with naturally producing antioxidants causes age-related diseases like cancer, heart diseases, and diabetes.

Apart from blueberries, there are other fruits, nuts and berries that fall into the superfood category, and you've probably heard of the acai berry trend which was touted as having even more antioxidant properties than the blueberry. Pomegranate and beetroot are also part of the superfood family with high levels of nitrate making them heart-healthy, lowering blood pressure levels and reducing blood clotting in human beings.

8.2 Through the Magnifying Glass

Certainly, eating a variety of fruits, nuts, berries, vegetables and, meat is essential for a normal and healthy diet. However, the notion is that by eating these superfoods in more excessive quantities, a person would be more likely to reap the health benefits of these foods. For example, by regularly consuming cocoa, a person can boost the health-promoting benefits of flavonoids.

Benefits of Adding More Fruits and Vegetables to Your Diet

- Fruits, nuts and vegetables contain electrolytes. Consuming these in abundance in your diet may help minimize the chances of getting fatigued and low energy

- A diet rich in fruits and vegetables reduces the amount of pesticides and chemicals that enter the body. It also reduces the consumption of animal by-products such as honey, thus reducing the destruction of honey bees, nature's primary pollinator

- It also reduces the number of antibiotics entering your system. Livestock production involves the use of antibiotics unless you purchase organic meat from free-range farms. Organically grown fruits and vegetables have no antibiotics in them

- Dieters have also reported clearer skin and better sleep quality

- Feeling overall lighter and energetic

8.3 Incorporating Fruits and Superfoods into your Daily Diet

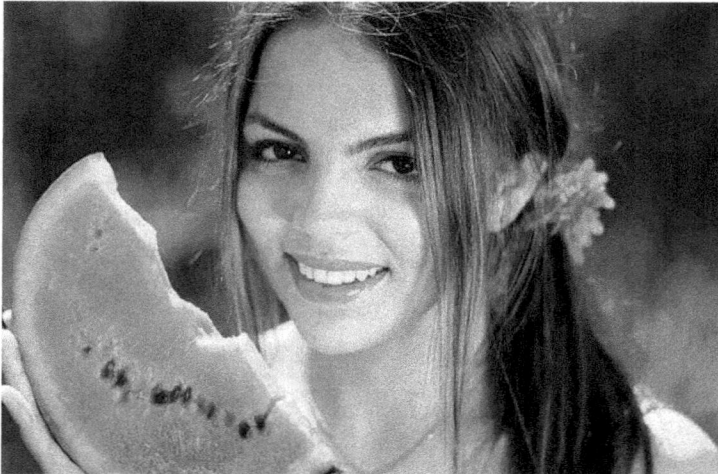

Most people tend to follow an unhealthy diet which reduces the amount of fruits and superfoods they consume or their diet consists of a select few ingredients- in other words; there is no variety. Variety is good for everyone. A combination of protein, carbohydrates, vegetables, nuts, grains, beans and dairy is essential for a healthy body.

But if your diet usually just consists of burgers and fries, fast food, soda drinks and fried foods, the likelihood of you eating anything that isn't brown or fried isn't very high. Too many people eat too many of the wrong kinds of foods simply because they either have not developed a taste for nutritional food or they aren't aware of the consequences of unhealthy food or just couldn't be bothered to alter their diet. Old habits are hard to break but on the other hand, it isn't entirely impossible.

If you are planning on revamping your diet and would like to eat the rainbow so to speak, then there are several ways that you can sneak in these superfoods to up the ante of your diet game.

Whatever diet you choose or the foods you want to consume, the general rule is to have loads of fruits, vegetables, nuts, beans, dairy, and omega 3- fatty acid-rich foods. Even if you do consume a good mix of all these foods, the challenge is to include more of these amazingly nutritious foods regularly into your daily diet. The bigger challenge is that not many people are big fans of superfoods' taste or texture.

However, according to Evelyn Tribole, co-author of the Stealth Health: How to Sneak Nutrition Painlessly Into Your Diet, working in power foods into your diet. It's all about eating the right recipes. Evelyn recommends considering the favorite foods you eat or the kinds of food that you eat regularly and figuring out how to add in some of these superfoods.

For example, if you love eating tuna casseroles or fish patties then make a smart substitute by opting for salmon as a seafood choice rather than tuna or cod or mackerel.

Another example is sneaking in flaxseed. It seems hard to think of how to include something that seems so non-versatile such as flaxseeds, but the thing is you can incorporate it into your granola for your morning breakfast or even muffins, soups and of course salads.

Conquering Food Biases

Our taste buds evolve as time passes. Think of how you loved sweet things when you were a kid. The urge to have very sweet food may not be as apparent when you get into adulthood. Also, predetermined ideas of foodstuff can also cause people not to try these foods before they can even taste it.

For example, when you were younger you probably hated broccoli because of the way it's been prepared. But certain foods can taste amazing if you cook it differently.

Consider giving broccoli a chance by changing the visual presentation of the dish. You can puree broccoli if you don't like the way it is. You can even roast, dice it, and shred it even. The objective is to change the appearance of your least favorite food so that you can consume it so that you can improve the odds of you eating by changing its appearance of texture.

One Step at A Time

If you want to make a healthy change and start eating more superfoods, remember don't overdo. The problem everyone makes when starting something new whether eating healthily, exercising, attempting a new habit or even learning a new skill is starting strong and starting hard but not having the momentum to get through or giving up because it's becoming too hard.

So even with changing your dietary habits, remember you do not have to eat all superfoods at one go or all the time. The idea is to start small and make dietary tweaks one at a time till it becomes a habit.

David Katz, MD says "Pick three things you can do each day, do it consistently, and it will become a habit," says Katz, co-author of the book Stealth Health: How to Sneak Age-Defying, Disease-Fighting Habits into Your Life without Really Trying. "It is the routines and habits that integrate good health into your lifestyle that will result in health and wellness."

One of the steps to take is substituting certain non-healthy items with smart alternatives such as choosing whole grains over refined grains. David Katz says, to start with easy replacing, so the benefits encourage you to create other substitutions and other changes.

Also, expanding your taste buds is a good idea. Sometimes, we may not be used to a certain food item such as chia seeds or bee pollen but keep trying to consume it. It may take some time before these new foods are added to your favorite food list. Research has shown that it takes up to 8 to 9 times for anyone to get used to eating a particular type of food before their eating preference is established.

Nutrition Tips from Evelyn Tribble and David Katz

Here are 15 tips to help you sneak in some fruits and superfood into your diet:

1- BLEND IT

Blending smoothies is an excellent idea to get those lesser eaten fruits and vegetables into your stomach. Smoothies are great for a snack, for breakfast and even for pre-or post- workout meals.

2- TOP IT

Using foods like tomatoes, leafy greens, nuts and even chia seeds as toppings for sandwiches and salads are an extremely easy way to upgrade your meal from average to healthy. Crunchy whole-grain cereal or flavorful granola is upgraded into an amazing, nutrition-dense breakfast with the addition of yogurt. Adding a bagful of spinach under your pizza toppings is a great way of adding greens to your meal.

3- PUREE IT

Pureeing food items is a great way of altering the texture, so it is much easier to eat. Pureed roasted vegetables make for a satisfying sauce as a side or even for dipping for chicken or fish meals. Pureed cauliflower is delicious as a topping for burgers. Pureed avocado becomes a great complement for salads.

4- STIR IT

Take a leaf out of Asian cuisine where vegetables are shredded before adding to fried rice, fried noodles, ramen or broth. Soups, stews, meatloaf, omelets, and quiches are ideal recipes where carrots, cucumbers, beets, garlic; avocado and leafy green can be added without compromising taste.

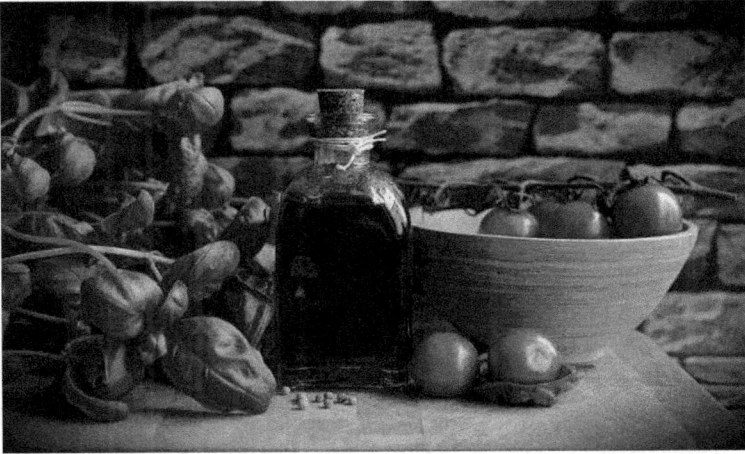

5- USE THIS NOT THAT

Substitute rice for cauliflower rice. Substitute dairy milk for almond milk in baking. Instead of beef or chicken, substitute it for tempeh. Substitute ricotta cheese with blended tofu, honey with agave syrup, and butter with olive oil. The options are endless.

6- BAKE IT

Everyone loves the smell coming out from the oven. Baking bread and muffins are a great way to upgrade it to a healthy option by adding bananas, blueberries, pumpkin, zucchini, carrots, and walnut.

7- ROAST, GRILL OR BROIL IT

Fruits and vegetables don't have to be eaten fresh all the time. Some roasting, grilling, and broiling elevates the subtle flavors of a variety of vegetables and fruits. For example, oven-dried cherry tomatoes give out an earthy flavor to any dish. Grilled jalapeno adds a rustic touch to any burgers, and grilled Portobello mushrooms are so good you can eat it on its own.

8- DIP IT

Make amazing dips with fruits such as an orange cream dip which is refreshing and delicious. A raspberry fruit dip is great as an addition to an afternoon tea spread. A coconut cream dip is a welcome on a hot summer afternoon.

9- EAT RAW

Of course, eating things raw is probably the easiest way to eat things. If you do not have time to make stuff, then cut them up and nibble it away. Celery on its own is great and can be eaten with minimal attention. So eat it while stuck in a traffic jam. Eating raw cucumbers, jicama or even a handful of goji and blueberries as a snack is a great way to increase your superfood intake by eating it raw.

10- BUY PRE-CUT

Sometimes, if you are lazy, purchasing pre-cut vegetables and fruits will increase the chances of you eating them. Also, purchase vegetable or fruit drinks such as cold-pressed pomegranate or cold-pressed celery and cucumber juice.

11- DISGUISE IT

Shredding things like lemon or spiraling zucchini and cucumber to add it into your pasta is an excellent disguise method.

12- SPICE IT

Herbs, spices, and vinegar are essential to the body and to flavor food. Make your healthy salads and soups come alive but simply adding oregano, basil, rosemary, and thyme can take a boring meal to a top-notch restaurant-level cuisine.

13- EXPERIMENT

Sometimes, changing the way you cook things will make you look forward to cooking the foodstuff and eating it more often. For example, eggplant is a great vegetable to cook Asian way by lightly sautéing it and just added garlic and soy sauce to create an easy yet delicious vegetable dish. Salmon is super delicious cooked with teriyaki sauce. Yam is always cooked as a steamed cake in Chinese cuisine. Turmeric, chilies, onions are a staple in Indian cooking.

14- BE ADVENTUROUS

Cooking on your own is a great way to pique interest and to try new things in your kitchen. If it doesn't turn out the way you want, learn from it and attempt to do it again. Start with simple dishes and work your way up by improving your cooking techniques and venturing outside your comfort zone. Try different cuisines and keep adding ways to add superfoods to your culinary adventure.

15- SEE HOW PROFESSIONALS PREPARE

With the multitude of cooking videos available online, it is easy to figure out the steps used to prep and cook an item like fish or chicken or beef. Watching how chefs and nutritional experts reinvent items like vegetables and nuts and seeds is an excellent eye-opener.

CHAPTER 9-

TRACK YOUR NEW HABITS

We talked about mindful eating, intuitive eating, explored intermittent fasting and even water fasting in helping you incorporate different ways to establish a positive relationship between you and food. So what's next? Part of successful anything- whether successful weight loss, career, goal accomplishments and target achievements, fitness goals- it all boils down to becoming accountable for your actions and tracking your progress. You need to track the changes you are going through and to see if it matches with the actions that you have taken. For example:

Action: You started intermittent fasting as a way of cutting down calories

Results: How do you feel after going through this for 7 days? Could your body handle not eating for 16 hours? How many consecutive days did you follow through with the fast?

Action: Your food rule is to drink 2 liters of water from the time you wake up till the time you have your breakfast.

Results: Did you notice that you had fewer cravings for sweet things in the morning? Did your water intake cut down your caffeine need? When we see the actions we have taken and the results it has procured, we are more likely to follow through a plan especially when we see positive results.

9.1 Goal Setting

Goal setting is really different for different people. But most goals fall into two major categories. The first are goals that we have a 95% chance of accomplishing, simply because we've done it before. The second category is the goals where there is a 95% chance of not knowing if we will accomplish them, simply because we've never done it before, but we would like to anyway.

There is numerous advice on how to do goal-setting right. So, in this chapter, we will explore not so much about how to set goals, but more on how to accomplish these goals. Our mind and our subconscious are set up to help us achieve goals that we sincerely believe are achievable. Here are some tricks that can help you in goal setting and goal getting:

Be A Dreamer, but Stay Motivated

Goals are materialized because every one of us is a dreamer. But to accomplish your goals, you need to do something about them and that takes self-discipline and motivation. Your first trick is a mind trick. Have a burning desire and a reason to achieve it. The path to achieving goals is filled with boredom, procrastination, anxiety, excuses, and difficulty. There will be so many times that you will try to talk yourself out of this goal. But to keep going, always remember the reason and the desire of why you wanted to attain this goal because this helps you stay on track.

Break into Smaller Goals

Break down your goals into mini-goals. Your brain probably knows you can't achieve enormous goals in an unrealistic timeline. So, when you create your goals, give it a 24-hour cycle. Essentially, create mini-goals. For example, if your goal is to eat healthy- don't tell yourself 'Ok! I'm going on a 30-day gluten-free diet today!'. No, it doesn't work that way. Instead of saying 30 days, tell yourself you will go for a 3-day gluten-free diet and move up from there. Your mini-goals must be reasonable, sustainable and attainable within your 24-hour period.

Work on something Everyday

The more you work on your habits and create a routine, the closer you are to achieving your goals. You would naturally take some time off but if you do not take the first 7 days or first 30 days of your working on your goal, you will never create the momentum you need to drive you till you reach your desired target. The first 30 days of a goal is crucial- it not only shows people you are serious; it also boosts your morale and drive to keep you going and sustain your goals well beyond your target.

Learn to adapt and adjust

As you go on daily achieving your mini-goals and working towards your bigger goals, be flexible. Be willing to adapt to changes along the way. Make your mini-goals slightly difficult if you deem them easy. Or if they become too taxing, then make them easier. The main thing is to remember that if it is too difficult, you might end up quitting. If it's' too easy, then you are pushing yourself. Find a middle ground that is decent for advancement each day. For example, if you have set your mini goal to do 30 pushups daily, by the time you are 2 weeks in your training, you might feel that you can do more. So challenge yourself and bring up the daily goal of doing 40 pushups daily.

Looking back for feedback, looking forward to reward

Feedback and reward are essential parts of goal-setting and goal-getting. On your

journey to goal-getting, be bold to request feedback from the people around, especially from the ones you look up to. Give yourself a little reward once a week or daily for accomplishing your goals. Rewarding yourself can be simple as putting a gold star on your calendar on the days you accomplished your goals, so something more elaborate like a dinner on Saturday night. This reward giving is positive reinforcement. These little things are good enough to tell your brain that you are doing something right.

Schedule Down Time

Slop time is when you do not need to focus on our goal. It is the time when you can allow yourself to cheat on it or not do it at all. We are humans and we are bound to do it anyway, so you might as well allow yourself that space to be normal humans. Allowing slop time is crucial because it prevents us from feeling dejected or get bored. Temporarily ignoring a goal for a short period (like during the weekend) is great to refocus your energy and do things better when you start the next week fresh. Just remember not to over-do it and don't make this a habit. Slop times are good if it is done once or twice a month.

Sticking to the small, boring stuff

Doing things on routine can get you bored. That is an undeniable fact. Achieving goals isn't about celebrating each time you complete a milestone. It's about sticking to the daily, small stuff no matter how boring it gets. Get the fundamentals right then make it slightly difficult the next day so you are constantly challenging yourself. Keep doing it again and again till it becomes a habit. When it becomes a habit, you'll realize that you look forward to doing it and it doesn't take that much effort as it used to.

9.2 10 Days towards Changing and Tracking Your Goals

DAY 1- FIND YOUR TOOLS

- Start the first day on a Sunday. The first step on the path to goal setting and tracking is to get you equipped with the right tools. Don't fret- you don't need major investments at this point. You only need the basic stuff- a notebook, a pen, poster board, and colored markers. Once you have these, take the rest of the day to think about what your goals are. Just think about where your life is right now and where you want it to or how you want it to be. What is your ideal life? Think about this in all aspects of your life- work, family, health and finance. Think about this and don't restrict yourself. This also about why aren't you leading a life like that now? Think about what skills you need to develop to get you to do your ideal life.

DAY 2- CREATE YOUR VISION BOARD AND TO DO LIST

- The path to successful weight loss (or any kind of success at all) is to write your goals down. Never rely on your memory to get this done. Whatever you have been thinking about the day before, right them down today. Create your mission statement. If your mission is to be happy and fit then write it down. If your personal mission is to run a marathon by the time you hit 30, write it down. If your mission statement is to volunteer your time as much as you can- then write it down. Write this down on your poster board with colored pens and motivating images or quotes. Place this vision board in a place that you can see every day.

DAY 3- CREATE A MORNING ROUTINE

- For permanent weight loss, start the day on a positive note. First Lady, Michelle Obama's morning routine is described as such in her interview for O, The Oprah Magazine in 2009"If I had to get up to take care of my kids, I'd get up to do that. But when it comes to yourself, then it's suddenly, 'Oh, I can't get up at 4:30.' So I had to change that. If I don't exercise, I won't feel good. I'll get depressed." Anna Wintour, Vogue Editor-in-Chief starts her day at 5.45am with a vigorous tennis match. AOL CEO, Tim Amstrong gets out of bed at 5 or 5.15 am to answer emails or sneak in a workout. As mentioned in previous chapters, starting small is always a good thing. So for day three onwards:

1. Start by waking up at least one hour earlier than your usual time.

2. Make your bed. Military training always places importance on soldiers making their bed perfectly. The reason is simply because you've accomplished one task in the morning!

3. Drink a glass of lemon water. Lemon water in the morning is known to boost energy and brainpower.

4. Do some light stretching to get your blood pumping and awaken your senses. If after this you feel like you are in the

mood for a run, go for it. If you feel like a 30-minute bodyweight workout- go for it!

5. Listen to your favorite songs during your shower. Songs give you a better mood to kick off the day!

6. Look at your vision board!

DAY 4- IDENTIFY YOUR ENVIRONMENT AND YOUR SOCIAL CIRCLE

- Today, it is time to observe. Once you have done your morning routine, head out to work. From the point of waking up till the time you get to work, observe the company you are with and the environment you are surrounded by. Make a note of all these things in your food journal or food app. Name the three people you admire most and describe the qualities that they have. What situations in your workday give you the greatest feelings of self-esteem and worth? In what areas do you feel you need to be more truthful and practice higher levels of integrity?

DAY 5- CREATE A MORNING ROUTINE AT WORK

Since we have done a morning routine when you wake up, creating a morning routine at work is also essential to your path of sustainable weight loss. Having all these different routines helps make your self-disciplined. A great app to use would be Coach.me and this can help you maintain and stick to your good habits. While at work, look around your workspace- is it in good order? Do you have things organized? Next, look at the people you speak with or have lunch with. How long do your meetings take?

What kind of person is your boss? When you get back home, reflect on all these items. See how you can improve your social circle and work environment to get closer to your weight goals by doing little changes along the way. Write down the actions that you want to take the next day. For example, if you have a fitness goal but you have a very desk-based job that does not allow you to move so much, maybe for the next few days, walk to lunch? Or do little exercises while at the desk? Do you spend so much time procrastinating by going through social media and Facebook that you end up snacking while browsing? Think about the things that you want to do the first thing you get into your office. Here's an example of how your morning routine at work can be:

- Switch on your computer. Drink a big glass of water.

- Read the newspaper or go through the day's news online

- Speak to your co-workers can catch up on work-related business.

- Check your calendar to see what you have scheduled the whole week

- Do tasks that require your immediate attention

- Reply emails

DAY 6- ORGANIZE YOUR WORKSPACE

Organizing your workspace benefits all aspects of your life. An organized workspace makes you look forward to work every morning. It keeps your mind uncluttered and it also helps with finishing tasks easily. Take some time off after your usual working hours to de-clutter your workspace. File papers, arrange books, organize your desk and drawers and most importantly- set this space up so it is conducive and encouraging. Paste a large calendar on your office wall so you can see what's ahead of you. Put up some encouraging words, quotes, and even images. Place a mini terrarium on your desk to brighten up the space. Having the color green or spending time with nature boosts our creativity. Research done by Cardiff University's School of Psychology shows that adding plants to a work area boosted a worker's productivity by 15 percent.

DAY 7- ORGANIZE YOUR HOME

Part of being self-disciplined is to de-clutter your life and since we did our office, it's time to work on our home. Clean up your home- sweep, mop, wipe and dust. Arrange your pantry and your fridge and get rid of all kinds of unnecessary and unhealthy foods. Scrub and clean floor tiles, bathrooms and sinks. Arrange your spices and boxes, pots and pans. Take the garbage out. You need to do this today, during the weekend so you start fresh the next week.

DAY 8- REFLECTION

It's Sunday again! Wake up late- you deserve it. Take it slow, have a cup of coffee, have a good breakfast, sit and talk with your spouse and children. Take this Sunday to meditate and look back at this whole week. What did you think needed improvement on? Were there areas that you can re-do again? Do you think there were better ways to do the things you did the whole week? Write down your thoughts in your self-discipline notebook to use them for the next coming weeks.

DAY 9- COMMIT TO SOME EXERCISE

After a whole week or organizing and de-cluttering your life and waking up an hour early, how does it feel? Do you feel like you have more time on your hands now? This week, you would feel a lot more energized and pumped up. Why not slot in exercise in your schedule? Exercise doesn't need to take an hour. All you need is 10 minutes of your day! HIIT workouts are great for those who want a quick workout but still burn calories. Commit to 10 minutes a day of exercise either in the morning or after you get back home.

DAY 10- BECOMING ALL YOU CAN BE

The only way to change your position in life right now is first, by changing yourself. Start your day in a positive way. If you think positive thoughts, you will experience positive events. Remember that no one else can change your life except yourself. Today's mantra is all about how your thoughts can become your words. Your words will become actions and your actions will become habits. Your habits shape your characters and your character becomes your destiny. Practicing self-discipline is a short-term pain that comes with numerous benefits in the long run.

CONCLUSION

You are at the end of the book! Along the way, did you try any of the steps, methods or plans described in this book? The very fact that you picked up this book already shows that you are one step into making careful and productive choices for your health and for your wellbeing. It takes a lot of courage to say admit that what you are doing right now in terms of dieting, eating, meal prep or your eating plans are not working for you or that you are doing it wrong.

Through intuitive eating, the relationship that we have with our food will hopefully be improved so we see food, not as a means to feed our emotional demons nor to suppress our feelings but rather sustenance to nourish our mind, body, and soul.

Intuitive eaters when eating, usually give themselves unconditional permission to eat whatever their hearts desire without feeling guilty. But here is where the mindful part comes in- knowing what to eat, how much to eat and when to eat so you get the proper nutrients in your body. Intuitive eating explores the awareness of the body's signals related to hunger and satiety and the decision to stop or go for more is entirely on yourself- you need to trust your body to tell your mind when, what and how much you want to eat.

You may feel like having that dessert but you know that you need to eat your veggies too. There is no guilt or regret when making choices because you trust yourself that you will make the right choice for your body. There is no fighting, no internal negative thoughts, no rewarding or punishing yourself.

You want to have a positive communication network with yourself, your body and your mind with the food you eat- this is a privilege not many

How Do You Know if Intuitive Eating Is the Right Approach for You?

The only way to know is to try it. You may have already attempted to practice intuitive and mindful eating before you even finish this book and that's great! So, ask yourself- how do you feel?

If you haven't already started, then here is another reason why you should give it a try. For one, you've done all other kinds of diets and eating plans, what's stopping you from trying this one?

Plus, the great thing about intuitive eating is not so much about a diet- it is not going to make you feel isolated or unhappy rather it benefits you in psychological and physical ways.

If you are already on a diet plan or an eating plan (such as intermittent or water fasting) then intuitive eating only helps you stick to the plan a little better without burnout because again, it puts you in charge of eating.

Can only eat at 1 pm after your 16-hour fast? No problem- I am doing this for me because I want to give my digestive system a break. Give myself a 20-minute break before I take another helping of lasagna? Nope, I want to dig it right now because it is delicious. No regrets.

Any day is a good day to start eating intuitively. It can even be the next meal you are going to take. Whatever you do, think about why you are doing it and what are your goals. Don't have goals? Well this is a good time to make it. Refer to the chapter where we discuss goal setting because it will help you define what are the outcomes you are looking for when it comes to your weight and it will also help you track the results. Remember that the reason you are doing this is because YOU OVERSEE YOUR BODY. You decide what and how you want to eat, how much and when.

I want to Stop Dieting and Start Intuitive Eating. How do I begin?

Well the fact that you've picked up this book is a great start as it gives you an idea of what intuitive eating entails. This book begins with 10 principles which you need to be aware of and know that is not another new diet fad. Think of this as more of a way of life, to reset our inhibitions with food and take control of eating.

After that, all you need to do is read up, commit to change your eating habits and make small tweaks in your daily life so you can be more intuitive and mindful eat time you eat and drink. It's that simple.

If you want to be more thorough, journal your food intake so you know what goes in, how you feel, why you ate certain things and how much and make small changes from there. You might also want to get rid of your scale and just trust the journey that you are on. Don't worry about the numbers going up or down-your aim is satisfaction with whatever that sustains you.

INTRODUCTION

Congratulations on purchasing *Intuitive Eating Workbook: A step by step mindful program for weight loss and* thank you for doing so. The following chapters will discuss how to develop a healthy relationship with food as well as how to strengthen your connection between food and your mind and body. If you're sick of counting calories and following fad diets, this book will introduce you to Intuitive Eating and how to use it to reach your weight loss and maintenance goals! Identifying what type of eater you are can lend powerful insight into your current relationship with food. Do you find yourself eating when you're bored and need to pass the time? Are you drawn to certain snacks during certain times of the day? Have you ever consoled yourself by eating food when you are having a hard time? If you're like most people, you've probably done all these things at some point in your life. We'll explore the main types of eaters and provide questions for each so that you can determine which types you identify with. This is the first part in truly understanding how to break negative patterns with eating, and to identify the beliefs you have around food.

Intuitive eating is a research-based eating style that we all have naturally at birth. It's through learned behavior and signals from society that we develop unhealthy relationships with food and hunger. Knowing the difference between real physical hunger and other types of false hunger can help us to rebuild that connection to our bodies' signals. We can start by not being afraid to allow ourselves to feel hunger! Only when we know we are truly hungry can we determine when we are truly full. Once we begin to recognize the signals we get from physical hunger we can work to provide our bodies with the nutritious foods needed. Think about the foods that you most enjoy? Why is it that you enjoy them? Is it because of how they make you feel? Is it because they taste good? These are important distinctions to make when it comes to discovering what will make you feel satisfied and not just full. With intuitive eating, you can eat whatever you want. Because most of us aren't used to this freedom, it can be easy to only choose those foods that we've restricted from ourselves. If you haven't taken the time to really venture out and taste different foods, now is the perfect opportunity. That doesn't mean that you must try everything, though it's certainly a lot more fun if you do, it simply means that you want to reintroduce foods into your diet that brings you joy or provide nutrients-no matter what they are!

Consider the foods that you typically consume on an average week or month. How many of these foods are considered healthy or nutritious? How many of them are considered junk foods, or unhealthy? When we come up with these associations it's important to examine where the connections are coming from. When examining your relationships with certain foods it's important to ask if you consider the food a "bad" food choice? Is it bad because it's damaging somehow for you to consume it?

Chances are, the foods we consider off-limits are put there because of their caloric content or associations with indulgence or even gluttony. For example, consider chocolate. Do we consider it an indulgence to enjoy chocolate? Why? Chocolate, especially dark chocolate, has been proven to have a host of nutritive properties and health benefits. If you enjoy eating chocolate, think about the times that you allow yourself to enjoy it. Is it when you are celebrating something? Is it when you're having a "cheat day"? How do you feel after you've consumed the chocolate? Guilty or disappointed? Exchange chocolate for any of your "guilty pleasures." Ask yourself these questions and determine where you developed your opinions about each food. This is an important step in intuitive eating because we are moving from a restrictive mindset that causes us to crave certain foods just because of the associations we give it. If we can have whatever we want whenever we want, we are more likely to make healthier choices over the long term.

When identifying your eating habits you will want to take an honest look at what drives you to eat. Are you eating on a regular schedule every day? Are you reaching for food as you run out of the door? Do you take the time to plan your meals, and make a point to sit down and enjoy them? In what ways can you improve how you are consuming your food? These are important questions to ask and answer in your food journal. What would you like to improve when it comes to the frequency, duration, and content of your meals? By doing this you may identify times where you are eating out of boredom, or when you are reaching for food when you are experiencing emotional triggers. Most of

3

us will turn to food to soothe our emotions at some point. This could be anxiety, depression, anger, loneliness, sadness, or any other emotion that causes you to seek out distraction and comfort. It's also important to keep a food log and make any notes about how food makes you feel. There are a lot of ways that foods can influence our moods and feelings, including causing both wanted and unwanted effects just from eating them. Most times when someone turns to food to comfort themselves, they then will feel guilty or disappointment afterward, creating a cycle that is very hard to break free from. When we can identify the ways that we are turning to food because of emotional reasons, we can begin to repair this relationship. This means allowing ourselves to experience our emotions fully, and work through them without food. Our food journals will help us find those foods that make us feel good, no matter what our emotional state is when we consume them. Mark these foods with a star or other symbol, so that you can easily see what you should incorporate into any meal plan you create for yourself.

Because intuitive eating doesn't follow any rigid plan or really have any rules, it will help if you can come up with your own routines and structure around what you will eat and the activities you will engage in. For example, if your goal is to lose weight and you're new to intuitive eating you may wish to set up an activity plan for at least three times per week. When it comes to creating your eating schedule, you can play it by ear. If you're the type of person that needs to eat only two or three times a day, great! If you prefer multiple, small meals throughout the day that's great too! There is no wrong or right way to go about this. Do what feels right for you and honor your hunger and body. Our hunger is how our bodies let us know it's time to refuel it. Making healthy food choices can go a long way when it comes to nutrition and overall health. Learning to make healthy, smart food choices is imperative to each of us. It's also important to choose foods that help us stay fuller, longer. When we do this, we decrease the habit of reaching for a snack or junk food because our meal wasn't satisfying.

Keeping our bodies active is also crucial to our health. If you've struggled with losing weight, it could be in part because of a lack of activity or even too much of the wrong activities. When we listen to our bodies and engage in those things that we enjoy, we can reap the health benefits while also avoiding those feelings of "having to" do the activity just to lose or maintain weight. When exercise is viewed as a punishment or negative experience it can be very ineffective. Consider the ways that you like to move your body. What things are easy for you, and what things would you like to be able to do better? Use that as your starting point when developing a fitness plan or exercise schedule to go along with your intuitive eating. Keep a journal that allows you to track your progress in ways other than simply weighing in on a scale. Getting rid of the dieting mentality can be a long process that involves many different factors. We want to recognize, reevaluate, and implement healthy habits in every way possible when it comes to our relationship with food and exercise.

Remember that this is a personal journey to repair your relationship with your body and food. You can meet your weight-loss goals with intuitive eating by creating a sustainable, nutrition-dense diet of the foods you enjoy the most. Follow this workbook and keep track of your progress in your journal as much as you can. Only you will be able to determine the progress you have made and hold yourself accountable for accepting your body and pursuing this journey of healthy eating! There are plenty of books on this subject on the market, thanks again for choosing this one! Every effort was made to ensure it is full of as much useful information as possible, please enjoy it!

CHAPTER 1:

INTUITIVE EATING

Since the early 1970's many weight management experts and health practitioners started the conversation surrounding emotional eating. There were programs built on improving health and promoting a healthy weight by implementing lifestyle changes and focusing on self-care rather than following diets. With Intuitive Eating, you quickly realize that you're the expert when it comes to your body and what you put into it. Essentially, intuitive eating is a style of eating that will increase your attitude towards your body image as well as towards food in general. It's extremely simple, just eat when you're hungry and stop once you are full. By trusting our bodies and the inherent intuition we have we can begin to pull away from all the dieting advice and fads. This means that we must relearn our bodies, and how to trust them. You can begin by noticing the differences between real, physical hunger and emotionally charged hunger. By focusing on the biological urges we receive when we need to replenish our nutrients, we can align ourselves to our bodies' signs and signals when we have physical hunger.

You can use this workbook to determine what type of eater you are, and how you can use this information to make plants and set personal boundaries to keep you focused on your well-being and health goals. This can also help you develop a healthy relationship with food, and why you make the decisions you do.

If you've struggled with losing weight it could be that you're not providing your body with what it really needs. It's important to understand your body-type and the foods that will work for you when it comes to feeling full. Crash-dieting and using pills or other drugs to help you maintain your weight is not sustainable. It's only by practicing intuitive and mindful eating practices that we can identify our current relationship with foods and what we must do to improve it. We must move away from this diet-mentality and focus on providing our bodies nutrient-dense foods and opportunities to move. Many people have hit the gym in hopes that they can burn off all the calories needed for weight loss but are disappointed when they don't get the results they hoped for. This is because many of us will ease up on those diets once we see some results or over-exert ourselves so much that we aren't consistently getting physical activity over time.

When we become preoccupied with the foods we are eating, we are more likely to binge on those foods we think we should stay away from when we "cheat." With intuitive eating, we move away from restricting foods so that nothing is off-limits. When we know we can eat whatever we want, we are less likely to seek out junk foods and snacks when we want to eat. When we eat intuitively, we become free from experiencing guilt or ethical dilemmas. In doing this we can honor our hunger, respect when we are full, and really enjoy the pleasure we get from eating.

Diet Culture

Healing the dieting mind can be an ongoing process that will cause us to reject the dieting propaganda that we're literally bombarded with from television and radio to food packaging, clothing, and many other products. Weight loss is a great benefit or byproduct that we get by adopting a healthy lifestyle, but it's not always an indication of one. While many people can improve their health by losing weight, too many people believe that they must lose weight to be healthy. There is a certain social phobia of being fat or looking fat. You are probably familiar with the way that fat people are shamed and even dismissed by the majority, no matter what that person's health may be. This is hard enough when it's coming from strangers or friends, but it can be dangerous when it comes to the medical community. It's common for physicians to immediately recommend weight loss as a solution to anything that could be ailing someone with a larger body before looking into other issues or forms of treatment. There are plenty of skinny that are unhealthy while plenty of overweight people are in great health.

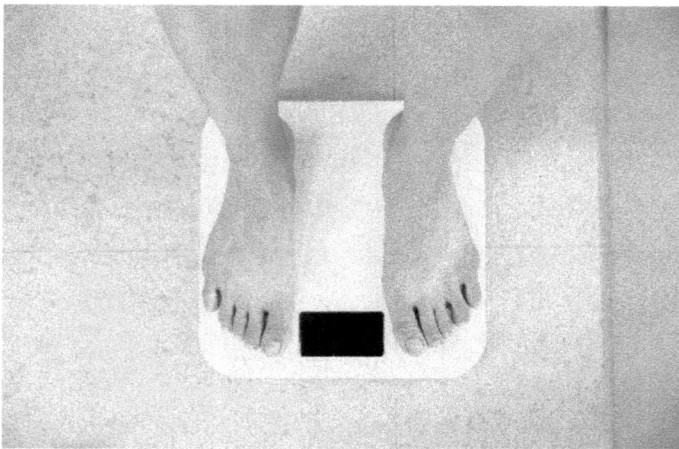

Common symptoms of the dieting mentality:

- Staying away from foods that you associate with being

"bad"

- Following rules of how much and what to eat, and when

- Anxiety surrounding making the wrong food decisions

- Guilt after consuming food

- Ignoring physical hunger

- The belief that supplements or other products are needed

- Feeling better or worse than others because of what you eat

- Shame or feelings of worthlessness due to body shape and size

- Exercise as atonement or punishment for eating

- Binge eating on "cheat" days

- Justifying what you eat to yourself and others

Diet culture essentially equates thinness to being healthy and having moral virtue. This is a toxic way of thinking that perpetuates eating disorders that are almost impossible to recover from without intervention. By reducing people to their body parts that constantly need to be worked on or fixed the dieting mentality causes many of us to attempt to achieve unattainable body types. Have you ever said, or heard someone say, "I feel fat?" Most times this is said when you feel bad or even gross. It's important to realize that "fat" isn't a feeling. It's a description that can be used in both positive and negative ways. If you mean that you feel that you've gained weight, you should consider how the dieting culture wants you to feel bad about it, and don't allow it to. Try to replace negative self-talk with more realistic phrases such as "I don't feel good about my body right now."

There is a huge profit to be made off our self-repression and hatred. The term "guilty pleasure" and "indulging" are concepts largely made up of this culture. This dieting mentality will have us believe that any time someone loses weight, it's a good thing no matter how it's achieved. This isn't true, as many people lose weight when they are depressed, are sick, or if they have an eating disorder. Since there is no way of knowing the reasons behind someone's weight loss, it's best to express that someone looks happy, or that they have a great outfit. That isn't to say there aren't people in your life that are on a weight loss journey that would appreciate some encouragement. You should check in with them and ask if and how they'd like for you to note or comment on their changes. The same goes for you. In what ways can the people around you support you on your journey? Would you rather that people not talk to you about it? It's not acceptable to comment on someone's body without their permission, and that includes you.

Food does not have an inherent morality. The belief that there are "good" and "bad" foods is a construct of dieting culture. Feeling bad because you've eaten foods that people associate negatively is not necessary. If you're trying to lose weight and are watching what you eat. There is no need to stress yourself out by designating certain foods as acceptable while others are off-limits. That food that you indulge in or consider your guilty pleasure could be someone else's favorite food that they eat normally-why would you want to bring them down? Now apply that to yourself. If you finish a big meal and then say something like "I'm so fat" you are only shaming yourself and anyone that's around you for eating. It means that you associate being fat with having little self-control, being overindulgent, and eating to excess. That's not fair to you or those around you, and it's certainly not kind. One of the most important things for the intuitive eater to realize is that there is nothing wrong with feeling full. If you have to say something, simply state that you're full, or that the food was good.

We've all probably been asked if something makes someone look fat. You may have asked someone that before concerning clothing that you think is unflattering. We want to move away from equating being fat with looking bad. This toxic diet culture is constantly telling us that we need to look as thin as possible. If you feel good in certain clothing, wear it. You can start to replace this way of thinking by asking "Do I look, and feel good in this?"

Cheat days are a common way for those on a diet to allow themselves food that they commonly restrict. When you say that you're having a "cheat day" you are telling everyone around you that what you are eating is somehow bad. Diet culture has led us to believe that we must have an excuse for eating certain things, but we don't need any reason other than we want to eat it. Many times even the strictest of dieters will completely go off the rails when it comes to their cheat days. By being strict all day or all week, they feel that they have somehow "earned" the right to indulge. What usually happens is that they then feel guilt or some loss of control as they attempt to eat all their favorite "bad" foods all at one time or in one day. Many will give up on their diets the next day thinking that since they've already eaten more than they wanted to there isn't any hope for them continuing. This is one of the largest symptoms of "yo-yo" dieting. Falling off the wagon, and then committing to doing it again. This is not a sustainable way to maintain optimum nutrition or overall health.

Another way that dieting culture rears its ugly head is when we hear someone say that they need to lose a certain amount of weight. If this is coming from someone that you consider healthy or fit, you may start to wonder how they view those that are heavier than they are. We must remember that the ways we talk about our bodies may affect how someone else feels about their own. No one else needs to hear about how far you are away from your "ideal" weight. You may have some experience with this, either hearing someone says they "need" to lose 5 pounds, or even guilty of saying things like this yourself. Try to replace this with phrases such as "I need to work on my mind/body relationship."

A powerful way to start dismantling the way diet culture has stolen joy from your life is to stand naked in front of a mirror. While we typically would immediately notice any areas that we do not like, we should honor our bodies and love those parts about us the most. Your body is your own. It can become easier to live in when you remind yourself that it's necessary to love the body as it is. Body positivity is arguably the best way to deconstruct the dieting culture from the inside out. We aren't alive just to watch what we eat and lose weight. Every type of body should be celebrated, but we are hardly exposed to different body types. This is especially true for fat bodies, disabled bodies, and the bodies of people of color. There are connections between fat-phobia and white supremacy, homophobia, and certainly misogyny. We must learn to realize that weight and body diversity has always existed and that those things are independent from health. We can improve our health by focusing on self-care and our habits-many times without any changes on the scale. The diet culture tells us that by being desperate to fit it, we will seek out those miracle cures that they sell us.

Remember, diets don't work because they are not meant to. Of course, when we fail at diets and losing weight we blame ourselves and seek out something else to help us. Our bodies are an inheritance from those who came before us, and it's also an ongoing act that we will play out every day. It's time to give yourself permission. To move through the world in your body, as it is, without the need or desire to change it.

With intuitive eating, we can come to understand our bodies well enough to trust them. There are no sets of rules or quick-fix diets. It doesn't matter how much you eat, or when or how. Intuitive eating is a lifestyle change, unlike dieting to reach a goal weight. There is a common misconception that dieting is a lifestyle change, but the problem with that is most people will regain any weight lost once they go back to their regular eating habits. When we switch from this dieting mentality we need to dig deep to figure out what happiness looks like for us. That happiness shouldn't be tied to a number that we see on a scale. There is no need to always be on a "plan" when it comes to eating and exercise. A commitment to listen to your body and respond to its signals while trying to do something physical every day is all that we need to sustain a healthy lifestyle.

Depending on where you are at regarding your weight loss journey, you may want to seek out a therapist to help you address your eating issues. It can be extremely beneficial to share your stories with someone that celebrates a healthy lifestyle without the constraints of diet culture. By starting to eat intuitively and separate yourself from this dieting mindset you can shift your focus and learn how those diets and weight loss strategies that you've tried in the past weren't beneficial to your health. When we focus on healing ourselves from the inside out this process becomes easier. Start with your emotional well being, and the ways that you talk to yourself.

Food Journal

With dieting, we are promised lots of different short cuts and magic tricks. This is not true for intuitive eating. One of the most powerful tools that you can use to change and improve your relationship with food is a journal. This is unlike any food journal you may have kept before. Instead of tracking your calories, amount of macro-nutrients, and the weight you will be tracking your favorite foods, emotions, cravings, and your thoughts. If you really commit to using a food journal at the start of your intuitive eating journey, eventually the things you are writing down will become internal habits. It's important to keep notes about any foods that cause you stress or anxiety. This will be important when it comes to recognizing your emotional triggers that can cause you to eat when you're not hungry. By keeping a physical record of the way you eat, you can notice your unconscious behavior and better understand it.

With intuitive eating, your food journal can help stop the critic and turn it into an explorer. This can help you reconnect with your already healthy eating habits naturally. It can help to keep you in touch with your physical responses to food as well as show you the ways that dieting culture is showing up in your life. Your food journal could be a simple notebook, or it could be a planner that you repurpose. It's important that your journal be accessible to you throughout the day-as we forget many important details if we can't write about them immediately. There are apps available so that you can take quick notes – but nothing will beat a pen and paper when it comes to really expressing yourself, and when it comes time for reviewing your journal.

Affirmations

If you're familiar with affirmations, then you know how powerful they can be for feeling better about yourself through simply repeating phrases. Using affirmations to help you improve your body image can provide you with that shift in how you feel about yourself. Make space in your journal to write in your own body-positive affirmations, or simply write down some of the following examples:

- I love myself, and my body

- I am happy with the way that I am

- I take care of my body by eating nourishing food

- I trust my judgment and listen to myself

- I deserve to be treated with respect and love

- I am worthy of love

- My body is a gift and it can do awesome things

- I trust my body and its wisdom

- I deserve to feel food and I enjoy feeling good.

- I am constantly growing and evolving

- My weight is not my identity

- My body is my responsibility, not anyone else's

- I love food that makes me feel good

- Food is not the enemy, and it has no power over me

- I thank my body for what it does

- It feels good to take care of myself

It's said that repeating affirmations first thing in the morning and again at bedtime can be powerful when it comes to positive thinking. Some people may choose to set reminders on their phone with an affirmation to remind themselves during the day. It's important that you use affirmations that resonate with you personally. Don't just write them down and forget about them. Repeat them, out loud. Try saying these things to yourself while looking in the mirror. It may seem silly at first, but your subconscious mind is always listening to the things you are saying to it. Be sure to surround yourself with as much body positivity as you can. Follow champions of self-love on social media, and only allow yourself to focus on others that show complete love for the bodies they live in.

As you practice these affirmations, you might just begin to convince yourself that you are perfectly acceptable just the way you are. This is just the first step in breaking away from the diet culture and moving towards a life of eating mindfully and intuitively. When you experience doubt or disappointment because you are falling back into your old ways of eating, revisit your affirmation page and remember that this will be an ongoing journey. We never stop evolving, and you can always update your affirmations to help you focus on trouble areas or to help remind you of how far you have come!

CHAPTER 2:

CATEGORIES OF EATERS

It's important to understand what type of eater you are so that you can identify what triggers you to overeat or make unhealthy food choices. Knowing what characteristics, you have as an eater can also give insight into how much you rely on your weight and appearance for happiness in your life. It is said that regarding those who are concerned with their weight, there are two main types of Eaters- Permitters and Restrictors. The restrictors are those that enjoy placing restrictions on the foods that they eat. This is typical because they enjoy the sense of control that they have when monitoring and selecting their diets. Permitters are the opposite of this, often preferring denial or ignorance when it comes to food. Intuitive eating can be beneficial for both types as it focuses on awareness and really knowing what your body wants and needs.

<u>Intuitive</u>

Someone that is conscious of their own hunger signals and mindful about their food choices is considered an intuitive eater. This is someone that doesn't experience guilt when they enjoy eating food, and there isn't a fear of overeating.

Questions you can ask yourself regarding Intuitive Eating:

- Do you eat when you're hungry and stop when you're full?

- Are you open to trying new foods and have a wide variety of foods that you enjoy?

- Can you enjoy a meal without feelings of guilt or shame?

If you can answer yes to any of these questions, then you are probably already familiar with eating mindfully. The intuitive eater will seek out the foods that they enjoy, when they want. It's by responding to the body's natural signals to eat and stop eating that this type of eater lives by. If you're not able to do these things quite yet, don't worry. This workbook will give you the techniques needed to start rejecting what you think you know about food and health and start seeking out a healthier lifestyle by giving yourself permission to eat what you need.

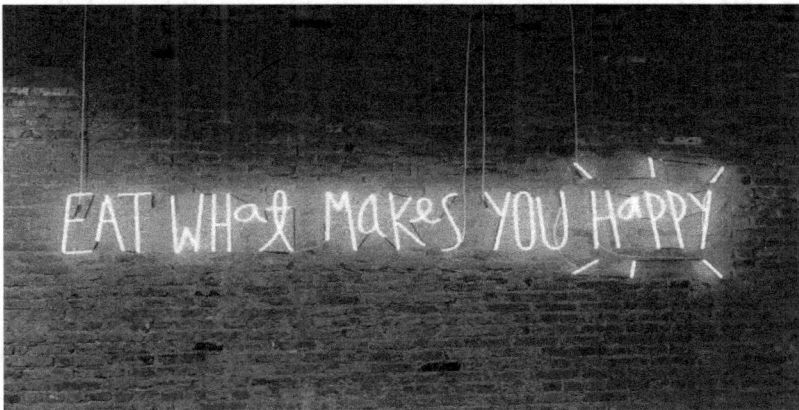

Restrictive

While this person is typically vigilant in reading nutritional labels, measuring out appropriate portion sizes, and is usually always on a diet, the restrictive eater doesn't get a lot of joy from eating. Because they have a constant need to examine what they are eating and when, they can become fearful of eating with others and even refuse to eat food prepared by anyone but themselves.

Questions you can ask yourself regarding Restrictive Eating:

- Are you often reading nutritional labels to see how many calories are in a serving size? This includes examining Carbs, Fats, and Protein quantity.

- Do you stop yourself from eating something you like because it doesn't fit into your daily plan?

- Do you consider yourself "off the wagon" if you eat something outside of what you had planned?

- Are you purchasing "diet" foods so that you can save calories?

Restrictive eaters are those that are on typical diets. While it's important to have some sense of self-control, we do not need to impose rules on ourselves when it comes to what food we are eating and when. With intuitive eating, we can learn to eat what foods we like when we are hungry for them. This can be a hard thing for a restrictive eater to achieve since there are many habits they rely on to tell them what is or is not acceptable to eat. When restricting ourselves from the food we enjoy we may believe we are making "healthy" decisions when we are depriving ourselves of one of the basic joys in life, eating!

Main Eating Types

Refuse Not

While none of us want to offend someone by turning down food that they have prepared, Refuse Not eaters find it extremely difficult to disappoint anyone when they are offered food, or invited to eat. This can lead to a loss of personal power as they are listening to others on how much they should eat instead of paying attention to their own hunger and fullness levels. This type of eater is usually unconscious about the food decisions they are making because they aren't paying attention to the physical intake of foods but rather the social interaction or circumstances surrounding the food.

Waste Not

We are all familiar with the term "clean your plate", but Waste Not eaters take this to a different level. This is someone that is constantly looking out for a deal that will get them the most food for the smallest price. This includes buffets and other places where food is unlimited or available in abundance. The Waste-Not eating type can have a hard time passing up any food offered to them. This type will typically ignore their body's natural signal that it is full and complete a large meal anyways. This can lead to always seeking out larger portion sizes because they start to believe they need that much food to feel satisfied.

Questions you can ask yourself regarding Waste-Not Eating:

- Do you seek out restaurants that have unlimited

quantities?

- Do you experience guilt if you do not finish all your food?

- Do you equate fullness with the quantity of food you eat?

- Are you more likely to purchase food because of the money you save rather than because it's something you want or need?

The waste-not method of thinking can be difficult to move away from, as many of us are raised believing that we must eat everything that is put before us. While we want to be careful to not be wasteful, we must learn to realize it's acceptable to turn down food or stop eating when we are finished. By listening to our bodies and finding out what portion sizes are best for us personally, we can start to only take the amount of food we know we need. When in doubt, start with less and once finished if you are still hungry for more, then get more!

Emotional

All the different types of eaters can be considered an "emotional" eater. A common theme in our society's messages about food is that indulging in certain foods will make you feel better emotionally. Too often we see these messages in television and movies as someone suffering from a relationship breaking up turning to a pint of ice cream or other "forbidden" food to binge on until those feelings are soothed. This is a dangerous cycle since turning to food to fill emotional needs will usually make us feel worse. To add insult to injury, once you are done binging and those emotional issues remain, we can also feel guilty for having eaten those foods, or for overeating! Emotional eaters tend to beat themselves up afterward for not having more willpower. This includes rewarding ourselves with foods that we have restricted ourselves from when dieting. This is also seen as emotional eating when we are running to these off-limit foods on "cheat days."

Eating food to cope with feelings is something most everyone has done at some point in their life. However, using food to soothe and even numb yourself can create a feeling of powerlessness. Emotional eaters tend to eat way too much, but not realize it until they are finished eating. If you find yourself celebrating with food, or soothing yourself with it, you may be an emotional eater.

Some questions you can ask yourself to determine if you are this type of eater:

- Do certain foods make you feel safe?

- What do you find yourself eating when you're stressed?

- In what ways are you rewarding yourself with food?

- Do you feel out of control around certain foods?

- Are there times that you eat until you're over-full?

- Are you eating to feel better about being sad, bored, or anxious?

Even if you are feeling powerless over food and emotions, you can make a positive change! You can put a stop to emotional eating by learning healthier ways to deal with your emotions, by conquering cravings and avoiding your emotional food triggers.

An easy way to determine if you are eating emotionally is by knowing when you have an urge to eat that is immediate, or overwhelming. True physical hunger will come on gradually and typically won't feel as dire for instant satisfaction. Physical hunger can be satiated by almost any food while emotional hunger typically drives us towards junk foods or sweets that can provide us with an instant rush. When we eat in response to emotional hunger we may be unaware of what we're doing and can eat entire containers of food without really enjoying them or even paying attention to the fact that we've done it. Even when our stomachs are full, emotional hunger can keep us wanting more and more until we are uncomfortably full. Since the hunger we feel emotionally isn't in our stomachs but rather our minds, we can be fixated on certain tastes, textures, and smells.

By identifying your own personal triggers- situations, feelings, people, and places that make you want to reach for those foods- you can work to gain your power back.

When we experience chronic stress our bodies produce high amounts of cortisol, a stress hormone. Increased levels of cortisol can trigger cravings for foods that provide a burst of pleasure and energy such as salty, fried foods, and sweets. If you have a lot of uncontrolled stress in your life, you may be turning to food as emotional relief. Another common cause of emotional eating is to use food to fill a void in our lives. By eating, you can distract yourself from uncomfortable emotions such as loneliness, anger, sadness, and shame. It's important to look for patterns in what drives us to eat certain foods and to overeat. Once patterns emerge, we can identify these triggers that drive the emotional eating response. We then need to create alternatives to food that can be turned to in times of emotional distress. This could be finding someone that you can reach out to when you're experiencing certain triggers. It could also mean finding other ways to distract yourself. The most effective way to deal with emotional eating is to become mindful of your emotions and allow yourself to experience them at the moment. With this, you can start to repair emotional problems that are triggering for you.

Unconscious

Also known as mindless eating, the unconscious eater typically lacks the mind-body connection due to habitually eating while doing other things. Of course, grabbing a quick bite to eat while running out of the door will happen to everyone from time to time. Unconscious eaters will usually eat anything that is available and always when they are engaged in another activity such as working, driving, watching TV, etc. This makes it hard to identify when one is full, or even hungry in the first place. When we mindlessly snack throughout the day without dedicating a time to enjoy a meal we can overindulge without realizing it. By taking the time to sit down to eat mindfully, we increase the chances that we will need less food to feel satisfied. Remember to take the time to savor your meal and retrain your brain to recognize that it's eating to meet a need.

One way that we can help to curb unconscious eating habits is by making certain foods harder to grab when we are in a hurry. By creating a bit of inconvenience to access foods that aren't as healthy we can train ourselves to opt for better food choices. Keep nutritious snacks and meals easily accessible while junk foods and other unhealthy choices should be more difficult to access.

Keep in mind that just because a food is labeled as "healthy" doesn't mean that it is. We should purchase food items based on the ingredients and nutrients that they contain rather than the health claims on the packaging. Mindless eaters can purchase healthier snacks in bulk so that when there isn't time to sit down and enjoy a meal, they at least know that they are making a better choice than usual.

Questions to help identify if you are an unconscious eater:

- Do you always eat something when you're out with friends or at parties?

- Do you always eat at the same time of day, even if you're not hungry?

- Are you too busy to eat, and find yourself rushing to eat between tasks?

- Do you eat well in the daytime but snack throughout the night?

While there are many different reasons that one might eat without realizing what they are eating or how much, it can easily be turned around. Determine what kind of mindless eater you are; emotional, social, pleasure, routine, or multitasking. You can then implement changes based on when you find yourself mindlessly consuming food.

Chaotic

Another person that eats on the run, the Chaotic eater tends to be overscheduled and lacks routine. This can cause them to skip meals frequently and to forget what they've already eaten or how much. Chaotic types will eat whatever is available and typically never plan out their meals. If you find that you have huge stretches of time between your meals, you could be overeating when you finally do eat. Chaotic eating can also be frequent snacking on anything accessible throughout the day. By doing this, we can cause our bodies to want more and more of those types of quick-fix foods.

It can be helpful to develop a routine for yourself if you tend to skip meals or if you're always eating while on the run. If you wait until you are already hungry before considering what you will eat, you will almost always go for the easiest or quickest food items.

Questions you can ask yourself regarding Chaotic Eating:

- Do you prioritize what you are doing overeating?

- Do you skip breakfast because you're in a rush?

- Are you eating a lot of take-out food because you're out of things at home?

- Do you eat all your meals at home, because you don't have access at work?

Additional Eating Types

Critical

Critical eaters will typically fall into the "all or nothing" mentality. Being dedicated to obsessive dieting habits can cause a person to only distinguish food in "good" and "bad" categories. This means they are either doing well with their diet or they aren't. When a Critical eater goes off the rails, they tend to allow their eating to spiral out of control since they've already messed up. They will then seek out new quick-fix diets such as detoxes and juicing to get themselves back on track.

Energy

This type of eater will focus on healthy snacks that can provide them with the energy they need for a task. While preparing with healthy food choices is recommended, you don't want to rely on these quick-fix snacks to provide most of your daily nutrition. Consuming these fast-acting carbohydrates that are typically found in even the healthiest snacks, can cause increased insulin production and lead to increased hunger levels. Spreading out your meals and providing smaller portions of the real thing in-between can be beneficial to energy eaters.

External

Visual cues drive this type of eater to consume foods even when they aren't truly hungry. This could be passing a shop window filled with cakes and sweets to television advertisement that shows appealing images of food. It's important to understand that just because you crave something, it doesn't mean that you are necessarily hungry and need to consume food. You can create distractions to allow it to pass, and if you're hungry-you can use that pause to consider finding a healthier alternative for your meal.

In your food journal create a section dedicated to discovering what type of eater you are, or what characteristics you identify with from each eating type. Ask some basic questions such as, if I was on a diet what would cause me to go off it? Would it be that the temptation of certain foods was enough to cause you to spiral out of control? Would something like a fight with your significant other be enough to send you directly to junk food? Do advertisements on food or seeing something while driving cause you to want things even if you're not hungry? Consider what you're most likely to eat for lunch tomorrow. Will it be something that you have planned or something that you decide on just minutes before lunchtime? Do you wait until the absolute last minute to eat? If you find yourself hungry between meals are you prepared with your own snacks or do you seek something from a vending machine or whatever else is available?

All these questions and more can provide powerful insight into how you are currently eating, and what you may need to work on to break away from your unhealthy eating habits. Notice the ways that you eat foods because you think you "deserve" them. Do you feel that it's more acceptable to consume certain foods only after you have been to the gym? You also want to make note of your energy levels. At what point during the day do you have the most energy and focus? Do you find that you lose focus as the day goes on? Once you've identified what type of eater you are, or the types that are most common for you, you can begin to change your relationship to food.

CHAPTER 3:

THE SCIENCE BEHIND INTUITIVE EATING

By relearning the basic instincts that we have for hunger and satisfaction, we can stop restricting food from ourselves and redefine what healthy looks and feels like for us individually. Do you know what hunger feels like for you? When you are full, do you know how to interpret the signals that your body gives? These are the main questions behind the science of intuitive eating. This means forgetting things such as "cheat days" and counting the foods you eat. It's essentially a dismantling of all dieting behaviors that you may have. Intuitive eating is a process of self-discovery. Because this is an ongoing process, you will constantly learn new things as much as you unlearn them. The first step when starting your own intuitive eating journey is to forget the diet mentality. This could mean that you start allowing yourself to eat sweets, load up on carbohydrates, or have as much as you want and need. You'll want to pick something you are restricting now and begin to unlearn it and challenge it. Once you've broken this old rule, you can begin to work on another-no matter how long anyone of them take you.

It's important to remember that intuitive eating is the anti-diet. By eating mindfully you can eat any food you want free from guilt. Many of us are drawn to diets that offer a quick-fix or easy way to lose weight quickly. The problem with a majority of these diets is that they restrict basic food and nutrients that our bodies want and need. Once we ease up on the restriction, any weight that was lost easily is gained again quickly. This causes more guilt and even shame as it creates a cycle of diet and gain, diet and gain. This method just isn't sustainable. We must reject society's message that any quick-fix diet will ever yield lasting results. You may want to go through your home and eliminate any dieting books or magazines that you've been drawn to. You may have noticed that when you deprive yourself of basic foods you can really feel that deprivation. When our bodies aren't getting what they want and need it can cause us to binge and overeat when we finally allow ourselves to have those items again. Many of us have unhealthy relationships with food because of these cycles. By designating a food as "forbidden" we subconsciously make them even more desired and tempting to us. With intuitive eating, we give ourselves permission to eat, unconditionally.

When you have no limitations you may be surprised to learn that even though you could eat chocolate cake and ice cream for breakfast, you probably won't because of how it will make you feel when you've finished. By learning how to question what you eat and why you want it, you can identify those ideas that you may need to unlearn. Intuitive eating includes practicing self-awareness, and that means really asking yourself if you really want something. If so, do you want it because you will really enjoy it in the moment or because it will feed your body with what it needs and wants for you at the time. This self-awareness extends into the middle of your meal. By pausing to assess how you feel and if you are still eating to feed the hunger you can begin to pick up on the satisfying responses you have. This can also help you identify when you are still eating because you are bored, stressed, or distracted.

One of the most important factors of intuitive eating is discovering your satisfaction factor. This includes the environment you are in, as well as the tastes and textures of your food. Truly understanding what feels good to you can be an ongoing process as your interests and tastes change. We must always stop for a moment and consider what it is that we really like to eat. What is it that feels good to your body? By asking yourself these questions and having go-to foods and meals that will bring you the satisfaction you can complete your meals and move on without guilt or worry. One easy method for doing this is to really focus on the first bite of your meal as well as one in the middle and the last bite. As you progress in your intuitive eating journey you can really place your awareness on any aspect of food that you're enjoying. You can begin to question what you enjoy about the good, from the taste, texture, and visual appearance.

Recognize and Change your Psychology

Some of us have deep-rooted psychological issues that cause us to eat at certain times such as when we are emotionally unstable, or anxious. There are also people that simply allow eating to get out of hand because they are distracted or not paying attention to what food you are eating, and how much. By increasing your mindfulness -with food and emotions- you can begin to sort out your emotional dependencies and habits surrounding eating. As you begin to identify the ways that overeat or indulge in unhealthy foods, you can search for other ways to nurture and soothe yourself without turning to foods. The first step in this process is to respect the body that you are meant to have. Too many of us strive for unrealistic expectations regarding how much we should weight, or what size clothing we should be able to fit into. Although intuitive eating is not a plan for weight loss, many will naturally lose weight once they can leave behind unhealthy habits with dieting and restrictions. By feeling good about our bodies and working to be the healthiest version of ourselves, we can easily obtain optimal wellness.

We can also feel more comfortable in our own skins by making a point to move our bodies on a regular basis. Many diets are accompanied by extreme workout routines that are also unsustainable in the long term. When we move away from searching for the perfect exercises to burn the highest number of calories in the shortest time, we can learn those activities that we enjoy. Just simply making a point to move our bodies every day can boost our mood and provide many health benefits such as strengthening the cardiovascular system and heart. While intuitive eating doesn't require any structure to follow, it can be helpful to develop your own routines when it comes to eating and exercise. Following standard portion sizes can be a great way to determine if you should prepare for a given food. Finding food that you enjoy from all the major food groups is one of the best ways for creating balanced meals for yourself. This also includes sourcing the highest quality foods that are in season and fit into your budget and tastes. Only you can decide the best times for you to eat, and how much. Eating foods that nutritionally dense and those typical "good for you" items will help you give your body what it needs for optimal health.

The true science behind intuitive eating is that when there are no foods that are off-limits for you, you are less likely to seek out those foods you think you shouldn't have. This also means it's less essential to continue to eat something until you are uncomfortable just because the opportunity has presented itself. By believing that you can't have something, you are giving that food more allure and power over you. By giving yourself permission to eat whatever you want, the foods still taste good, but you've removed that sense of urgency you have in eating them.

Identify your Habits

It is recommended that you start a food journal. You'll use this journal to perform a current-state analysis in later chapters of this book. For this purpose, you can make a list of the foods that you consider "off-limits" when you are and are not dieting. You can define all the reasons that food is on this list-from what it contains to any connotations that it carries with it. Next, make a list of all the foods that you are typically able to eat on any given fad diet. What makes these foods good? Why should you be allowed to eat as much as you want on any given food? Take your time in doing this and make note of all the foods that you enjoy. Make a new list of your favorite foods-incorporating items from both of your previous lists. Consider when you allow yourself to indulge in any items from the "bad" list. Do you only turn to those foods when you have given up or ended a round of dieting? How do you feel when you consume them? Do you typically eat just enough to really enjoy those foods or are you feeling any guilt or shame after eating them? Your food journal is for your eyes only and should be used to help you identify what you're withholding from yourself and what you find yourself really craving. It's said that the body craves what it needs. While we can interpret our bodies' signals incorrectly, we can develop this connection so that eventually we know what to feed our bodies when we receive these different signals.

If you are dealing with a serious eating disorder, you should seek medical advice. Many times those with eating disorders cannot properly regulate their intake of food on a biological level—and turning to intuitive eating may not be the best move. Once your biology is under control, then you can find intuitive eating to be helpful.

It's important to realize that intuitive eating isn't only "eating when you're hungry and stopping when you're full." If you're at a birthday party and everyone is enjoying cake, you may indulge even if you're not hungry at the moment so that you can celebrate as well. Sometimes you might find that your schedule is full, and you'll need to eat something before you're hungry because you know you won't have the opportunity to eat later.

CHAPTER 4:

NATURAL HUNGER

We all experience hunger differently, but there are ways to identify patterns in our individual symptoms. The hypothalamus is the part of our brain that partially controls hunger along with hormone levels, blood sugar levels, and how empty the stomach and intestines. When our body tells our brain that the stomach is empty, we feel true physical hunger, which is a normal sensation. Hunger is different from Appetite. The desire for food can be caused by seeing, smelling and even just thinking about it. Appetites can cause us to continue eating even when we are already full and stop us from eating even when we are physically hungry.

Many of us are under the impression that we should never experience hunger. While we do not want to prolong hunger symptoms that can cause us to lose focus and level-headedness, it's normal to experience moderate hunger up to four times a day! This physical hunger be is a sign that our metabolism is working correctly and that it's burned off everything it could from your previous meal. By waiting for the hunger symptoms to be signaled, you are listening to when your body needs you to refuel it for the coming hours. Even when we plan out every meal to provide the exact amount of nutrition that we want, we can still overeat because we're not listening to the natural queues that our body gives us when it's time to eat.

Physical hunger symptoms are typically below the neck and occur several hours after eating a meal. These feelings typically fade once you are full, and a feeling of satisfaction replaces them. Some additional hunger symptoms that everyone may experience:

- Stomach growling, or rumbling

- Lack of focus and concentration

- Nausea

- Easily agitated and even irritable

- Light-headedness or dizziness

- Feeling empty

Our physical hunger symptoms are the body's way to keep us in balance. We can embrace this and use it to our advantage! Try eating a balanced breakfast using the recommended portion amounts. Pay attention to the amount of time it takes before you start to feel the physical sensations of hunger. You should notice these hunger symptoms within three to four hours after eating this breakfast. If you can go five or more hours without any symptoms, try to cut the portion size back a little the following day. We should become mild to moderately hungry every three to five hours after every meal to remain in balance.

It can take the body up to 20 minutes to communicate to the brain that we are full. If we are distracted when we eat or eat a large amount of food very quickly we may never be able to recognize the signal that we are full.

On the other hand, emotional hunger is typically felt above the neck and is unrelated to time. Even after eating, emotional hunger can continue and often that eating causes feelings of guilt and shame. So how does the Intuitive Eater mentality compare to a Diet Mentality? Those with a diet mentality will typically ask if they deserve the food they want while an intuitive mentality would ask if they want it and if they are hungry for something. Where someone with a dieter's mentality would view food as the enemy or describe a day of eating as "good" or "bad" the intuitive eater will ask if it tastes good and knows that they deserve to enjoy what they eat without feeling any guilt. This carries over to the way we view exercise. A person with a diet mentality will focus on the calories that they burn and feel a sense of guilt if they miss a workout, the intuitive eater will focus on how that exercise makes them feel and enjoys how energizing it can be. Finally, the way that we view our progress is quite different between the two mentalities. While a person with a dieting mentality will focus on how many pounds they've lost, and what other people think of their looks the person with the intuitive mentality will recognize their inner body cues and focus on developing a greater trust with themselves and their food.

Mindful Eating

We can become more familiar with our body's internal queues by simply focusing on what we are eating and when! Concentrate on the present moment so that you can really taste and savor the food you have. In doing this, you will use all your senses and inherently become more aware of your choices. There are many ways that we practice mindful eating:

Eat Slowly- Make the decision to eat your food more slowly. This could mean that you chew your food more than normal, or by taking smaller bites. You can use your non-dominant hand to eat or put your fork down in=between bites. The goal here is to take time to breathe between bites and really taste your food.

Clean Up- Ensure that your dining area is clear of items that can take your attention away from eating. This includes your cell phone, papers, and other items. By creating a clear space where you eat, you can keep yourself focused on the experience of eating and reduce mindlessly indulging while you are preoccupied.

Take a Seat- Try to limit the things you are engaging in while eating. We may all enjoy sitting down to our favorite television shows while we eat dinner, but are we really paying attention to our internal queues when we do this? If you can focus only on eating you can quickly increase your mind/body connection with hunger and satisfaction.

Assess the Situation- You can do this by thinking before you start to eat. Determine your hunger scale before deciding if it's time to eat a full meal, or if a snack will suffice. Doing this will help you identify those times when you might be eating to fulfill a need other than physical hunger. Before you eat, find out where you are at on the hunger scale so that you can avoid overeating. It's okay to leave some food on your plate, so stop when you're satisfied!

Get a smaller plate- Downsize the plate you use for main meals. Doing this can create the illusion that you are eating more food than normal because the plate is completely full. If you need more food once it's finished, then get it! This is just one way we can move away from eating with our eyes. The quantity of food we consume should only be to provide enough for us to feel full and satisfied. When we eat beyond that point, we are doing so to excess. By eating from a smaller plate we start with smaller portion sizes. You may realize that you are able to feel full with much less food than you are currently used to.

Awareness- Find your number on the hunger scale before determining what you will eat. Are you really hungry or just wanting to eat? Honor your awareness by providing your body with what it needs. It could be that you're a bit dehydrated and a glass of water can alleviate some of your symptoms. By increasing your awareness of your body's signals you will be able to intuitively provide it what it needs.

Focus- Eliminate distractions so that you can focus on your food. Imagine that you will be writing a review of your meal, what details do you start to pick up on that you wouldn't normally? Take your time when enjoying your food. Notice the textures, smells, tastes, and every detail that you can ascertain. By completely focusing our attention on the foods that we are ingesting, we can derive further satisfaction from it. How well do you chew your food? Try to chew your food completely before swallowing it. This technique can help us to appreciate different characteristics of the food as well as give our digestive system a break. If we make a commitment to fully chew our foods, we will inherently become more mindful of how that food makes us feel.

Principles of Intuitive Eating

Reject the Mentality of a Dieter

Any diet that offers quick success with ease should be thrown out. There is no such thing as a quick fix. It's important to move away from the vicious cycle of "on again" "off again" eating habits. This includes getting rid of any hope that there is a new and even better diet just around the corner. Only when we can get rid of those hopes and expectations that we associate with dieting can we rediscover how to eat intuitively. Consider your relationship with eating and exercise. Start to take notice of all the ways dieting is pushed on us every day. In your journal, write down the ways that you can start to break old ways of thinking when it comes to food. Make note of the restrictions and opinions that you currently have and compare them to your ideal.

Honoring Health

Choose foods that make you feel good and are good for your body. The foods that you consistently eat are what matter the most. Having your favorite junk foods or indulging in sweets at a party isn't going to suddenly cause a nutrient deficiency-it's what you're putting into your body over time that matters. It's quite possible to achieve optimum health while eating the foods that you like. Take an assessment of your current state of health. Do you consider yourself healthy? What would you need to feel healthier, or to be in better health? It's important to accept yourself for where you are right now. If there are changes you need to make regarding the food you eat and the amount of physical exercise you get- then now is the time to commit to doing just that. Understand that your overall health has much more to do with your lifestyle and habits than it does with simply the foods you eat.

Honoring Hunger

If you provide your body with proper nutrition before you experience excessive hunger you can build a much healthier relationship with food. Turn your focus away from moderation and move it towards giving your body what it needs. This means providing your body with adequate carbohydrates, proteins, and fats. When we don't receive those basic staples in our diet it can trigger a drive to overeat. With dieting, we often will ignore our hunger or prolong it because we've already eaten, or we know we will be eating again later. This can have negative effects on your body since physical hunger is a sign that the body needs caloric intake or certain nutrients. When we prevent our body from receiving what it needs it can go into survival or starvation mode where the signals that typically burn the energy we provide are switched to burn off needed components like protein. We can honor our hunger by listening to our bodies and providing adequate nutrition when it is called for. In your journal, make note of the ways that you are and are not honoring your hunger currently. When your stomach growls or you start to feel physical symptoms of hunger, what do you do?

Exercise

Instead of focusing on the calorie-burning effect of a certain exercise, or the amount of time you spend doing it, notice how it feels to move your body and the benefits you get from it. It can be easier to find motivation from the enjoyment we get from doing something than simply making ourselves do it because we feel we need to. If you have a hard time finding physical activities that you enjoy it could be because you've only ever done those things to lose weight. Consider the exercises or the physical activities that make you feel good. We can use exercise to work out our feelings and emotions while reaping the health benefits. This could be anything from a simple walk around the block to group exercise or swimming. It's important that you find physical activities that you enjoy that you can engage in often. If you have physical limitations due to health issues or disability, you may want to discuss options with a healthcare professional. Simply sitting and standing repeatedly or taking the stairs instead of an elevator can be considered exercise. Choose those activities that are empowering for you. What makes you feel stronger? What gives you energy and a sense of renewal?

Body Acceptance and Respect

Having realistic expectations for your body and ideal weight is important. We shouldn't expect to weigh the same as someone that has a completely different body frame than we do. Loving our bodies for what they are and what they do for us is one of the best ways to develop a healthier relationship with food. This is a hard concept to grasp for most of us who have been inundated with dieting propaganda since we were children. If you are overweight, you are probably no stranger to being treated differently by peers or feeling that you aren't as good or worthy as those who are viewed as thin or healthy. We must learn to accept and honor our bodies for what they are, and what they do for us. If you are not happy with your current weight, ask yourself why.

Is it because you are dealing with health issues that are related to your weight? If so, then you can use intuitive eating to create a sustainable change in your relationship with food. If you're not happy with your size or shape because of any other reason, I urge you to reexamine your feelings around this.

Our bodies can do incredible things and practicing self-love and acceptance we can develop a healthier self-image. It can be a powerful exercise to consider some of the times that you were most happy. Now think about your body during those moments-how were you using your body? Did it matter that you weren't completely happy with how you looked? Do you feel that you can be happy regardless of how much you weigh? Create a section of your journal to reflect on these questions. What do you need to truly appreciate your body and what it does for you? In what ways are you honoring your body right now?

Making Peace with Food

Eliminate words like "can't", or "shouldn't" when it comes to the foods you eat. This can lead to binging behavior. This includes getting rid of the policing you have with food-including stopping when you hit a calorie amount and now when you feel full. We need to accept that calories are what makes food what it is. There are plenty of "diet foods" that eliminate the natural make-up of food and replace them with dozens of additives and preservatives. We essentially lose most of what made that food what it is in the first place. Think of the "reduced-fat" or "sugar-free" foods that you commonly see in the marketplace. Most of these take away the natural properties of the foods and substitute them for man-made chemicals, some of which are harmful to us. While it is wise to limit our intake of high fructose corn syrup and other man-made ingredients that are added to foods typically produced on a mass-scale, we don't need to eliminate them from our diets completely.

This also includes reexamining processed foods. While there are many processed foods that are full of chemicals and preservatives such as frozen dinners and meat-based items, the term "processed" can be applied to many natural foods as well. Even lentils and grains can be considered processed if they are in any way manipulated from their original form. The diet industry is not only good at demonizing foods based on their caloric content, it's also good at being reductive of foods that are mostly nutritious. With intuitive eating, we must learn that all foods are acceptable for us when eaten when needed and not to excess.

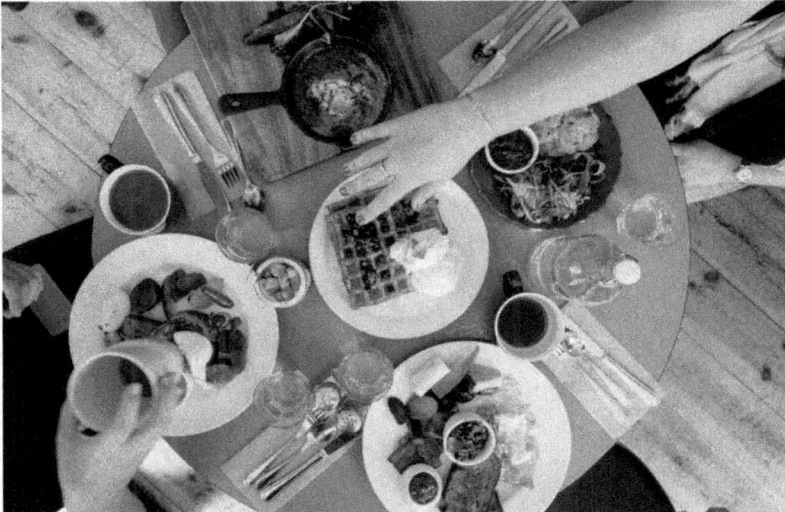

Discovering Satisfaction

This includes discovering and listening to your body's signals when it is full. When we eat the foods that we really want it becomes much easier to decide when we've had enough. This is more than just being full. We only will feel satisfied with what we are eating if we enjoy the food we are consuming. Think about a time that you may have been dieting where you eat plenty of food that you don't particularly care for. You probably ate it because it was "healthy" for you, or because of its caloric content alone. When you were finished with the meal, you were most likely already looking forward to your next meal because the food you ate didn't satisfy you. When we can learn to eat foods that we enjoy based on their taste, texture, smells, etc., then we are more likely to be satisfied with what we eat.

Your food journal is important for discovering those foods that you know are satisfying. You can keep notes on those foods that you enjoy, and those that you don't care for, and even dislike. That way, when it comes to planning out your meals or cooking, you have a list of foods that you can work with to provide you the best opportunities for nutrition while achieving satisfaction.

By incorporating these principles into your daily life we can practice the "Health at Every Size" approach to life. When we focus on weight-neutral outcomes we can experience improved eating habits, body image, and self-esteem. To recap, we need to learn to recognize our own hunger signals. With practice, we can pick up on them again. Avoid letting your hunger level drop below a 3 on the hunger scale if possible. When we get that hungry we are more likely to eat more quickly and make unhealthy choices. We want to allow ourselves to experience some hunger between meals. Hunger pangs are a natural part of life, and if we are reacting to them by eating-they are there to help us.

CHAPTER 5:

REVOLUTIONARY HEALING STAGES FOR THE INTUITIVE EATER

Do we really need to diet? Any food rules that are restrictive that we place on ourselves can be considered dieting. Some of us will require special diets based on health-related issues, and if you are following the guidance of a physician you should continue to do so. When we approach eating with feelings of guilt and shame we are doing so with a "diet mentality." Many times we may find that we are putting ourselves on a diet, however unintentionally, by setting rules around food. The diet industry is a multi-billion-dollar industry that in many ways hopes that we fail on our diets so that we will continue to purchase their products. The myth that people fail diets because they lack willpower is just one of the many psychological factors that continue to drive people to yo-yo dieting.

There are biological factors such as the hormonal, metabolic, and neurological changes that all contribute to us failing our diets, and why dieting will not help us maintain any weight loss. This includes us finding foods that we restrict ourselves from more tempting and appetizing that they would normally.

Hormonal changes include increasing those that make us feel hunger while decreasing those that help us to feel full. When we diet our metabolism slows down as our bodies use calories in the most efficient way. When our bodies are running on fewer calories we can find that we consume an excess that in turn gets stored as fat. These are just some of the reasons that over 90 percent of all people will consider their dieting unsuccessful. Even if weight is lost in the short-term, most people will regain everything they lost and usually will put on even more weight!

There is also a lot of psychological reasons that dieting doesn't work. When we tie happiness to an external achievement such as weight loss, we assume that it will automatically change our lives somehow for the better. The problem with this is that most people will find that their lives remain the same as before. Many people want to be "thin" because of the meanings that they have assigned to thinness. Some allow this desire to become obsessive, believing that it's something that they can control so they exert total control over themselves when it comes to their weight. No matter how hard we may try, we cannot control our external environment by manipulating our weight.

The Revolutionary Stages

Trust. This can be the hardest part, trusting the process. Eating intuitively is an ongoing process that can take some time to get used to. You will experience challenges along the way and setbacks that you'll have to overcome. When you have made the decision to pursue eating intuitively, you've already made progress towards your goal of improving the connection you have with your body. It's important to consider the journey just as important as the destination. Trust in yourself and the choices you make.

Support. Breaking away from the dieting mentality and moving towards intuitive eating can come with a lot of doubt and second-guessing. Find those people in your life that are supportive of your efforts. When you have at least one other person that you can trust to discuss your journey you can lean on them to get you back on track when you're having a hard time.

Relearn. A large portion of eating intuitively is unlearning those unhealthy habits you've picked up from the dieting culture. Our bodies also need to relearn to trust us. We can rebuild that trust by listening to and responding to our natural signals for hunger and fullness. In doing this you increase the ways you are showing your body that it can trust you and develop that mutual trust between you and your body.

Rules. Throw them out. Make a list of all your past and current rules around food, and practice breaking each one. This includes any rules you have around what you shouldn't or can't eat. Make note of how you feel before, during, and after experimenting with breaking all your food rules.

Practice. It's going to take a lot of work to re-establish the connection you have with your body while rejecting most of what you've learned from the dieting mindset. We must keep practicing, especially when we are full of doubt about whether that inner voice that leads our intuitive eating will ever come back.

<u>Fear of Food</u>

While there is an actual medical condition that people can

experience causing them to literally have a fear of certain foods, we are referring to a form of an eating disorder that is caused by excessive dieting and restrictive eating. This is commonly experienced by those who always carry their own food on them when they suddenly run out, or when they are not prepared at a certain point during the day. The technical term is called orthorexia, and it's caused by having a vice-like grip on only eating healthy foods. This can also be caused by the elation and high that one can experience from losing weight. They can begin to control their diet in ways that aren't sustainable and new and more strict restrictions come into play. If you decline an invitation to dinner because you know what's on the menu or stop going to new places because you can't trust the food choices-you may be developing an unhealthy fear of food. If you think that you are already suffering from this fear, you may want to seek out a specialized therapist that can help you work through your anxieties and the root causes of your fears around food.

We all must work to love and accept our bodies for exactly how they are at any given time. With this self-acceptance, we are more able to achieve optimum wellness. There are many people that are considered overweight that are much healthier than others that are thought to have an "ideal" body. Weight is not a good measure of someone's overall health. Therefore it's so important that we shift our mindset from weight loss to healthy living so that we can incorporate healthy habits and practices to improve our health overall. Multiple studies have shown that by simply changing our behaviors when it comes to health and nutrition, we can make huge improvements whether we lose any weight or not. If weight loss is your goal, you'll want to do some soul searching to determine the reasons behind this desire. There are plenty of healthy reasons for wanting to get in shape and improve cardiovascular endurance, and weight loss is usually a welcome byproduct of these efforts.

Naturally Balanced Diet

When we focus on giving our bodies the nutrients it needs to function properly we can adjust our mindset away from counting calories and watching the scale. Instead, we can look at the quality of the foods we eat, and the way they make us feel. It can be a tricky business to create a properly balanced diet for you personally, especially when there are so many different sources of information pulling you in different directions. Essentially most of your daily calories should come from fresh fruits and vegetables, whole grains, nuts and legumes, and lean proteins. Most adults need anywhere from 1500-3000 calories every single day just to maintain their current weight and energy consumption needs. Each person will have different needs based on their gender, age, and levels of physical activity. You also need to consider your body frame size, and how many calories you typically burn while at complete rest. This isn't to say that you need to count calories every day, it's simply a reminder that you need to provide your body with what it needs. When we do not provide our bodies with the nutrition it needs to work effectively we run the risk of fatigue, disease, infections, and overall poor performance.

Essential Food Groups

Below we will explore the food groups that are essential to

creating any balanced nutrition plan:

Fruits

We should aim to incorporate fresh, in-season fruits to provide nutrient-dense sources of natural sugar. While this is better than choosing foods that have added sugars, fruits can be high in sugar overall. If you are a diabetic or have other conditions that you monitor, you'll want to opt for fruits that have a lower-sugar ratio. Fruits are incredibly nutritious and should be eaten daily. Make a list of your favorite fruits and be sure to try new fruits whenever you can!

Grains

Whole grains that are prepared using the entire grain, as well as the hullm provide much more nutrition than refined white flour products. Most of the nutrition in grain lies in the hull which is removed when the grain is refined. These grains are high in fiber and will help to keep us feeling full while we benefit from a wide array of health benefits.

Vegetables

Fresh vegetables should be the primary source of essential vitamins and minerals in any nutritional plan. You can choose vegetables by their color to be sure you are getting different minerals and nutrients from a wide variety of options. What are your favorite vegetables? What vegetables would you like to try?

Protein

There are many natural sources of protein, though many people who diet will limit themselves to eating only chicken or by consuming high-protein shakes or bars. In addition to most meat, beans and nuts are also great sources of natural protein that is packed with other beneficial nutrients and fiber. Protein is one of the "macro" nutrients, meaning one of the nutrients our bodies need to function. Diets high in protein typically burn more calories throughout the day for energy use.

Oils/Fats

While they should be used sparingly, good fats and oils are essential to any nutritional plan. We should limit the number of deep-fried foods that contain an abundance of "empty" calories, we can find many options such as olive oil or flax that can offer omega fatty acids and other nutrients. Fats are another macronutrient that is essential in our diets.

Dairy

There is much debate surrounding dairy, and if it's essential for nutrition. While dairy is one of the best ways to obtain Calcium and Vitamin D, there are other ways that you can find these nutrients in naturally occurring foods. That doesn't mean do not consume dairy if you do not enjoy it, but that there are alternatives to getting these nutrients if you do not already consume dairy foods.

While there are many other foods that you may enjoy and want to continue eating, you should try to incorporate something from each of these food groups every day. Intuitive eating isn't just about eating what you want, it's about eating what your body wants and needs.

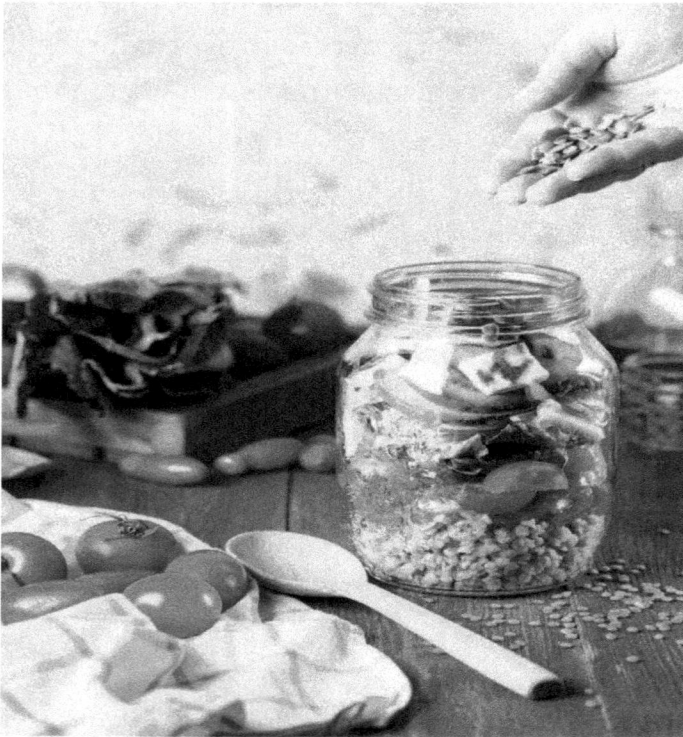

Hunger Scale

Determining where you are at on the hunger scale before you begin to eat can go a long way in helping you understand when you are truly hungry and when you are full. Below is a quick guide to breaking down the hunger scale:

1. Think of this as your "tank is empty." If you are at a zero, you have waited too long to eat, and you may be dizzy or irritable.

2. You're so hungry that you'll basically eat anything. Restaurant menus are quickly scanned to find something that will give you a quick fix.

3. You're preoccupied with your hunger and are willing to eat anything that's easily accessible.

4. You have a strong urge to eat and are experiencing several hunger symptoms. This is the "physical hunger number" that you want to designate for most of your meals.

5. At this number, you're starting to get a little hungry. You know you'll be hungrier soon, but you can wait to eat.

6. This is a neutral number, where you're comfortable being neither hungry or full.

7. You're satisfied but could eat more even with the sense of food in your belly.

8. At seven, your hunger is gone. You know that if you stop eating now you will remain satisfied for the next few hours.

9. You're very full and begin to feel as if you've overeaten.

10. At nine you're getting uncomfortable and need to loosen your belt because you've overeaten.

11. You've eaten too much and are now very uncomfortable.

In your food journal, make a space to write in where you are at on the hunger scale before you eat anything. Leave a space at the bottom of your meal notes to include where you were at on the hunger scale once you finished your meal. Understanding your signals for fullness and satisfaction are just as important as those signals that cause you to eat. If you have any meals where you are going past a 7 when it comes to fullness, you are eating to excess. If you find that you eat to excess multiple times a day or week, you'll want to reevaluate what you need to feel full.

Reflect on your journal in the weeks and months to come to see the progress you've made when it comes to the number of times you are eating past a 7 on the scale. Also, keep track of how often you are waiting to eat (3 or below) when you know you are hungry. Most people who are used to dieting will hold back from eating until they are extremely hungry. When we wait to eat we are more likely to overeat and indulge in foods that are quick and easy instead of healthy options. Use this hunger scale to help you keep track of how you are eating now and to provide yourself with a basic guideline on what your body is telling you, and when.

The intuitive eater must learn to embrace their bodies. Healing from disordered eating and the diet culture can be difficult, and we must work on starting the healing process.

Do some research on pro-body positivity and Health at Every Size. There are plenty of people out there that have rejected the dieting mentality and are helping others to stop dieting and reclaim their lives.

Stop engaging in any diet talk. This could mean simply not entering into conversations that are focused on dieting and exercise. When you hear people talking about counting calories, eating clean, being "bad" because they gave in and ate something sweet, etc., just remove yourself from the situation. There will be times when someone comments on your body such as "you look like you've lost weight" or "you look good, have you lost weight?" that you will inevitably have to deal with. Remember, your body isn't open to commentary from others. You have just as much value as a person whether you are overweight or not.

Start looking at images of real people that celebrate their bodies for the way they are. If you follow any accounts or friends that are constantly promoting weight loss, posting before and after photos, pushing dieting fads, etc., stop. Unsubscribe to anything that is not going to help you on your intuitive eating journey.

Quit trying to fit into clothes that are too small for you. Many times we will keep clothes that we don't fit into in hopes that we will lose weight and be able to fit into them again. Get rid of your "goal" clothing and buy yourself something that fits you now.

CHAPTER 6:

REMODELING EMOTIONS

Our emotions are a physiological and mental state that relates to our behaviors, thoughts, and feelings. We all experience emotions differently because they are such subjective experiences. When it comes to emotional eating, we're referring to any time we eat for reasons outside of physical hunger symptoms. This type of eating can be caused by both conscious and unconscious intentions and typically leads to eating in excess. Considering the obesity epidemic that is predicted to only increase, and the amount of eating disorders that we are aware of- one would think that we have lots of information concerning emotional-eating but we don't! There is actually very little in terms of research regarding emotional eating and the psychology around it. We are, however, starting to understand that our specific moods such as joy and sadness have been found to have strong effects in the responses to food choices, quantity, digestion and more. When we eat to satisfy our physical hunger, we should find that experience as rewarding and even pleasurable. Emotional responses to food start at infancy where babies respond to sweet and fatty foods that can ease crying and other behaviors, and these responses change as we age. There are multiple chemicals and neurotransmitters that are engaged every time we eat-and that can cause a real dependency on the effects we get from food.

While our emotions can have a powerful influence over the foods we choose and our eating behaviors, the same is true in reverse. Our eating behaviors can directly influence our emotions as well. This can be a dangerous cycle for some, as this emotional eating can relate to overeating, seeking out sweet and high-fat foods. We can see food affecting behavior in the change of mood that happens before and after eating a meal. Imagine that you're very thirsty and don't want anything but a huge glass of ice water. If you can't get that, it can have a negative effect on your mood and emotions. If you can get the water, your attitude and emotions can be greatly improved once you have quenched your thirst. We must be careful about how we are allowing our hunger and eating habits to contribute to our moods when we are able.

There is a system that was developed to help measure overeating from emotional needs based on some of the most common emotions: anger, tiredness, sadness, happiness, loneliness, and anxiety. This is a self-report form that is used over the course of a month to track how many times you experienced those emotions and how often they were connected to food and eating habits. It can be a difficult process to track emotional eating habits because of how these triggers can be so different from person to person and even from day to day. It's been found that most often, those who fall victim to episodes of emotional eating do so at home when they are alone.

Common Emotions as Triggers

Below, we explore some of these more common emotional triggers and implications of each:

Stress

One of the most common emotional triggers related to eating, stress can be a "catch-all" for all other emotions that we experience. We could have an emotional reaction based on the stress we have in our life, and we can be stressed out from experiencing other negative emotions repeatedly. Even further, we can cause even more stress when it triggers emotional eating as the cycle seems endless. Any feelings of physical and emotional tension can be described as stress. It's the natural way our bodies react to challenges and demands. While this response can be beneficial in short bursts and durations, it can be quite detrimental to our health. If you are experiencing a high amount of stress in your daily life, the chances you are eating emotionally is high. Studies are starting to show that stress-induced emotional eaters tend to favor comfort foods that come with guilt after it's been eaten.

There are lots of different steps we can take to manage our stress so that we are no longer a victim of it. We want to be as active as possible when finding ways to manage stress. This includes physical activity, and spending time on hobbies. Spend time with your favorite people and loved ones. Practice relaxation by participating in meditation, yoga, and deep breathing. When we pair these activities with getting plenty of sleep and providing our bodies with nutritious foods it can help alleviate the symptoms we experience from stress. If you're unable to control your step or have reason to believe that something other than stress is causing you distress you may want to seek out professional help. Therapists and counselors are trained to identify stress responses, help you find the sources of your stress, and help you develop new ways to cope with your stress.

Depression

There are associations between depression and a diet that contains high amounts of highly processed, and refined foods. So not only are we turning to foods that are bad for us when we feel depressed, those very foods could be causing us to feel that way! Some emotional eaters will binge eat to numb or dull their hopeless and sad feelings. Others may turn to food for comfort unconsciously, but the cycle of overeating or eating foods that are high-calorie, fatty and sweet can keep you from gaining control. On the opposite end of this emotional eating spectrum are those that become depressed and refrain from eating much food at all. Both extremes are causing our bodies to become nutritionally unbalanced, and intuitive eating can help you realign with your body's requirements.

While we all will experience feelings of loneliness and sadness from time to time, those of us that deal with chronic depression should seek professional help. If you are feeling hopeless or that you cannot control what you are doing from day to day, it can be helpful to talk to someone about your experiences.

Boredom

One of the least helpful reasons that we eat, boredom can cause us to fill time by eating food. Generally, we eat out of boredom when we are not physically hungry and after a few bites we decide to keep eating even though we realize that it isn't really satisfying any need. The chemical dopamine is a powerful factor in eating when we are bored. Since we can trigger our dopamine by eating, it's common to indulge simply because we have nothing better to do. What can we do to prevent this from happening? First, we can get rid of boredom by doing something that can take our mind off things. If you catch yourself eating out of boredom, attempt to fill that void by doing something you enjoy such as journaling, cleaning, or exercising. Try pouring yourself a big glass of water to hydrate instead of eating. Hot tea is also a great way to feel that you're indulging in something without the negative health benefits of overeating or eating when you're not hungry. If you've just got to give in to the feeling, try to eat something that is nutritious so that you can avoid any feelings of guilt later.

Anger

When we are upset or angry we may feel the need to hold these emotions in and avoid conflict. This can lead to suppressing feelings by eating or using food as a distraction. If you deal with bottling up your emotions and holding back expressing yourself by eating, it can lead to negative health side effects in addition to weight gain and lack of proper nutrition. Finding healthy outlets for your feelings of anger can go a long way. Exercise is a great way to express your feelings since it causes you to physically move and work out those emotions. Others prefer practicing relaxation and mindfulness techniques that can help relieve feelings of anger and helplessness.

Happiness

Eating when you're celebrating or when you've experienced success is something that we all indulge in from time to time. Since eating is one of the most sensual pleasures in life, it makes sense that we can derive happiness from eating just as much as we can celebrate by eating when we are already happy. Even the act of preparing and cooking our food can be a source of happiness. Those with eating disorders can derive a sense of happiness from restricting their food, or when their body is in a starving state. When we find a food that makes us feel good, such as those high in sugar, our bodies will naturally crave that feeling again. This can be dangerous if we are relying on food as a source of happiness and not nutrition.

With intuitive eating, we can learn to celebrate our happy times and deal with our struggles in ways that are healthy. No matter what your triggers are for emotional eating, it is wise to allow yourself to experience the emotions fully. Take a few moments to accept how you are feeling, whether that's stress or happiness or anything in between. We can train ourselves to rewire our habits by substituting a new choice. Sometimes we can get stuck in a pattern of eating such as every time we sit down to watch a movie, or when we pull a long study session. One easy way to break a pattern is to do something out of the norm such as brushing your teeth when you feel the need to grab a snack.

Chances are you won't want to eat junk food right after you've brushed your teeth, so it can be a powerful way to take your time and decide if you want to eat because you're hungry or because you're reacting to an emotional trigger.

CHAPTER 7:

EATING ROUTINE

When we think of eating routines and meal plans we probably associate them with dieting. Typically when we are planning our meals we are doing so because we are trying to limit ourselves to a certain number of calories or watching what we eat somehow. When it comes to intuitive eating we think of meal planning and eating routines to discover the foods that bring us the most satisfaction, and those that we know make us feel good. If you're already used to making yourself eat at certain times and in certain quantities, it may be easier for you to determine how to change those habits for the better. If you've never planned out your meals then you're probably used to eating on the run or eating out frequently during the week. By taking the time to purchase and prepare our foods we strengthen our relationships with those foods. It's true that you can find enjoyment from cooking the foods you and your family enjoy, and you don't need to be a chef to make a great tasting meal. If you're not used to cooking your own foods, now is a great time to experiment. We all have certain foods that we consider our "favorites" and foods that we know we really don't like. Use that as the starting point when creating a meal plan for yourself. This doesn't mean that you need to plan out every little thing that you eat, but it can be helpful to have at least one or two of your meals planned for the day. That way you don't have to think about what you're going to eat or where because you've already got something in place.

A great place to start is to consider your breakfast meals throughout the week. Are you typically grabbing something quick as you run out of the door on your way to work? Try to wake up a little bit earlier so that you have time to prepare something for yourself. Imagine what your morning would look like if you were able to take the time to cook yourself a fresh meal rather than eating in the car or grabbing fast food. How do you think you will feel when you get to work knowing that you've eaten until you were full and that you've eaten foods that you really like? Do the same thing with lunch. Make time at the end of the day to prepare your lunch for the next day. That way, you can use your lunch break to eat that prepared meal and have time to fit in some activity.

Most of the time when we think of meal planning outside of dieting, it's the dinner meal. Planning in advance what you will prepare for dinner is one of the best ways to save money and provide nutritious meals for you and your family. With a little time and effort you can cook fresh meals every day of the week while focusing on strengthening your relationship with food. Be adventurous and try out recipes that are new to you. If you're not used to cooking, seek out advice from family and friends that like to cook. Most people are happy to share their favorite recipes or even show you how to prepare their signature dish. If you don't have a signature dish of your own, work on finding one! While it's normal to not have time to prepare complex recipes and luxurious items every day, it's very easy to find easy to prepare meals that you like. Crockpot meals are a huge time saver for those of us that work long hours or have commitments after the work day. There are dozens of cookbooks for using a crockpot, and most meals can be prepared in advance and even frozen so that you can simply place them in the crockpot before leaving for the day. It can be a huge relief to come home at the end of a long workday to a meal that is ready to eat instead of having to start a recipe from scratch.

No matter how you currently eat most of your meals, there is always room for improvement. Try to replace at least one meal a day with something that you've prepared for yourself. With a little practice you may find that you prefer the foods you cook over anything that you can find at a fast-food restaurant. And if you find there are times that you would rather eat out at a restaurant or skip preparing dinner and just grab something quick, you can do so without any feelings of guilt. That's the beauty of eating intuitively- you can provide yourself the food you want when you want it. There is no reason to deny yourself something you love just because it's not the healthiest thing you can eat. Enjoying a taco or burger from a great restaurant once a week or so isn't going to make a huge difference in your overall nutrition.

Analyzing your Current Food Routine

By examining what you are eating now, you can make

changes where necessary. The best way to analyze your eating behaviors is by tracking what you are eating. This will help you identify patterns in food choices, and in portion sizes. While you're tracking you can also discover areas where emotions and other triggers are involved in your eating. With intuitive eating, you're making a lifestyle change and identifying your current eating plan is a great way to jumpstart your journey.

Be careful to stay away from monitoring and tracking what you eat with a dieting mindset. You want to keep a record of your food only to determine where you are at- not to judge yourself for how you eat. In a food journal you'll want to document everything that you put into your mouth for at least a week or two. Create sections for the following; time of day, the food or drink you consumed, how it was prepared, where you obtained the food, how much you ate, how you were feeling, who was with you, where you ate, and any physical activity that you had that day. If manually keeping track is not feasible for you, you may want to use a computer or find an app that can track things for you.

Once you have tracked for a couple of weeks you can compare your records to see if any patterns emerge. If you have multiple problem areas, you can pick one to start with and work on it first. Common problem areas will include the following:

High amounts of junk food or processed foods

Low amounts of fruits and vegetables

Low amounts of whole grains

Low amounts of meat and fist

High amounts of full-fat dairy

Calorie dense snacks between main meals

Skipping meals

Eating on the run

Habitual and emotional eating

Compare the times of day in your chart and notice if there are certain times of the day that you are reaching for any of these problem areas. There could be certain people that come through your life during the day or week, stressful situations, or simply boredom that can drive our unhealthy eating habits. As you start to find patterns in the foods that you eat, ask yourself why you choose those foods. Is it because they taste great and make you feel good? Is it because they are cheap and easy? In what ways would you like to change the way you currently source your food? What grocery stores do you shop from, and why? Are there other stores that you've considered shopping at but have prevented yourself because you're not sure how to prepare your own food? Are there ingredients that you've wanted to work with but haven't because of inexperience? All these factors should be considered when you are tracking the ways that you eat. Are you on a strict budget because you're feeding a family? Are you single and have a hard time shopping for food because it goes to waste? Take stock of where you're starting from so that you can map out how to get where you want to be. Think about how you'd like to eat throughout your day. In what ways can you make changes to help you get there? It may be as simple as planning ahead or finding a meal that your entire family loves.

Now that you've identified your current eating behaviors it's time to set goals for yourself to ensure your success with intuitive eating. Keep these goals small, and achievable- don't restrict things from your diet, simply incorporate those things you know your body needs. If done correctly, this will be the last time you start any eating plans!

Goal Planning

Creating goals surrounding the way you eat foods can be easy. Maybe you simply want to increase the number of vegetables you eat per week. You might want to simply drink more water or incorporate more variety to your drinks. Come up with a plan to help you achieve these goals as well. If you want to eat more vegetables, you must make them accessible to you. It can be difficult to come up with goals when it comes to foods while moving away from the dieting mentality. Try to be very specific and stay away from general statements such as "I want to eat healthier foods" or "I want to eat less." Put specific parameters around each goal. This could be "I want to try a new vegetable this week" or "I want to eat fish for at least one meal today." By doing this you can easily achieve your goals which will provide you with the motivation to set larger goals for yourself. Don't set goals for yourself just so that you can award yourself with certain foods. With intuitive eating you don't have to restrict anything from your diet, so food is no longer a reward. You can indulge in any food that you like at any time, so work on shifting your mindset from restriction/reward to simply finding those foods that you love most and how you can improve your nutrient intake at every meal.

Below are common goals, and tips for succeeding with your goals.

Portion

If you noticed from your food journal that you're eating way too much, not finishing your food, or feeling like you must finish your plate even though you aren't hungry anymore- you may want to set a goal on consuming healthier portion sizes. This is a good goal to start with since it's easy to achieve. Set a goal such as using a smaller plate to serve your food on. That way, if you finish the plate and you're still hungry you can always get more. This will also help you to pause for a moment and allow the signals of fullness that may have already been sent to catch up to your brain. On the other hand, if you're used to limiting the amount of food you eat to control caloric intake, allow yourself to eat as much as you'd if you stop when you're satisfied.

A great place to start with portion sizes is by looking at a recommended serving on a snack or food that you like. Start with the recommended amount and once you are finished, determine if you want more or if that was enough. It can take some work to recognize your body's signals when it comes to being satisfied. If you find that you're not satisfied after eating more than one or two servings, you may want to examine what's driving you to eat more. Is it because you're still hungry? If so, the food you are currently eating may not be providing your body with what it really needs now. If you're not still hungry but you still want to eat, it is probably being driven by your emotions.

Snacking

You may have noticed patterns with the snacks you eat and when. You may choose to set a goal that improves the quality and/or quantity of the snack foods you consume. Any snacks that can help you incorporate foods from the major food groups should be considered a great way to get the nutrition you need. Look for ways that you can increase the amount of fiber, healthy fats, and/or proteins so that your snacking can help sustain your hunger levels for longer periods of time. A goal could be as simple as including one snack a day that has an added nutritional benefit. Many people that are on a diet will be very strict during the day but let it all unravel once they get home and start to snack. It's also common for chronic dieters to limit themselves from snacking throughout the day. It's perfectly fine to have a snack between meals if you need energy or a bit more fuel to keep you going to your next meal. Provide yourself with snacks that are nutritious and with those that you enjoy. Snacks don't just have to be junk food such as chips and sweets. Nuts, trail mix, cheese and crackers, fruit, veggie sticks, beef jerky, and a host of other foods can be great snacks. Find what you like and in what quantities.

Eating Enough

Many of us do not get the nutrition we require, but because we're so full from all the empty calories we consume that we don't realize it. If you've found that you're not consuming enough food because you're skipping meals, or simply eating small meals while on the go, you may want to develop goals around how many times and the amount of food you're eating. An easy goal to set for yourself could include making time to sit down and eat at least two to three times every day. When we consider the number of calories we need to eat just to maintain our natural body weight, it's important that we are not restricting ourselves to that number of calories daily.

We want to be sure that we are providing our bodies with enough calories. The basic guidelines for this are around 2000 calories per day for a woman and around 2500 calories daily for men. This will depend on your current weight, height, age, and current activity level. The more active you are, the more calories you require to maintain your current weight. There are many different calculators available online so that you can figure out your required minimum. It is true that you can consume more calories and still sustain weight loss efforts if you increase your physical activity.

Water

We could all benefit from drinking more water on average. This is also an easy goal to achieve since water is mostly very easily accessible to us and it's free. Besides food, water is the most important thing you can provide your body. Symptoms of mild dehydration can include headaches, changes in mood, sensitivity to pain, nausea, dizziness, and more. Since we are made up of 60% water, we require quite a bit of water every day. We're all familiar with the rule of "drink 8 glasses per day." This equals 2-liters or a half-gallon! If you're looking to lose weight, increasing your water intake can help by reducing your appetite and increasing your metabolism. It is said that consuming water a half hour before you eat can help reduce the amount of food you eat overall. Drinking cold water can also help as your body will need to use more calories, or energy, to heat that water to your body temperature.

Plain water may not be your favorite drink, and it's important to remember that we are consuming water through mostly every drink and even some foods. Tea is an obvious alternative to plain water, and certain varieties such as green tea provide us with numerous other health benefits. Foods such as soups, fruits, and vegetables can contain large amounts of water and can be counted towards our daily intake as well. Lettuce, celery, cabbage, cantaloupe, zucchini, and watermelon are all made up of over 90% water!

When we set a goal as general as "drink more water" we set ourselves up for failure since we're not holding ourselves accountable for doing it. One easy way to drink more water is to set a goal for water consumption such as only drinking water with one meal, swapping at least one drink a day for water, and so on. If you are setting a goal to drink more water every day, make it easy for yourself by keeping a reusable water bottle at your desk or in your bag. Set a reminder for yourself on your phone or use an app that can spur you to drink a small glass every hour or so. A great way to start is by drinking a full glass of water as soon as you wake up for the day and drink another right before bedtime.

Intuitive Eating Meal Planning

When you plan meals with intuitive eating you move away from basing your choices on calorie content, and towards variety and options. Most people who plan out their meals do so with a dieting mindset and food restrictions. You can make intuitive eating and meal planning work together by considering the foods that bring you pleasure. You can also work to change your mindset by considering meal planning as meal "preparedness." When you are prepared to feed yourself it allows you to easily respond to your natural hunger signals with confidence. It also challenges you to include a wider array of food options for yourself to really relearn what your body wants and needs. You can work to provide nutrition by simply adding a vegetable to each meal when you prepare them.

It's important to consider how much time you will have to cook the foods that you have purchased. Meal planning can be helpful when you want to incorporate nourishing foods more often. While a meal plan is something you would follow on a diet, meal preparedness and planning is a process that you lead by your preferences and experiences. That means that it's completely flexible and you can relax knowing that you can change and adapt without feeling that you must stick to any certain plan to be successful. You can empower yourself to make better decisions when it comes to nourishing your body. This can also provide temporary structure that can make switching to intuitive eating a bit easier. When your intention behind meal planning is to help you focus on nutrition and to eliminate distractions, it can be very useful when getting in touch with your body's signals and needs. This will also help you have a plan in place for those times when you need to prepare something quickly. When you have the foods you know you want to eat on hand, it can help prevent throwing something together quickly and then binging on other snacks mindlessly just hours later.

Choice vs. Calories

When choosing what foods to incorporate in your meal planning, you want to avoid evaluating your food based on its caloric or nutrient content alone. That is a dieting behavior that can limit our focus on what foods bring us enjoyment and pleasure. With intuitive eating, you want to remove judgment from the foods you choose. Remember, it's okay to try new things and find that you simply don't like them. This can help to remove the pressure of feeling like you always must prepare meals at home from scratch. If you don't have time to cut and prepare fresh fruits and vegetables, opt for canned or frozen varieties!

Remember that you don't want your meal planning to be too rigid. With intuitive eating, planning your food is a strategy we use so that we are making rational food decisions when we are hungry. It is more about meal preparedness than it is about making yourself eat only what you have planned. If you've tried meal planning in the past, but failed, it could be because it was taking up too much of your time or you were too consumed with counting the calories for each meal. While some of us prefer to enjoy a lot of the same foods every day, others prefer a wide variety.

Additional Strategies

Shop Smart. Purchase foods that last longer when possible. If you're not pressured to eat certain foods before they go bad, you have more time to choose foods that you really want. Vegetables that are hardier such as cauliflower, carrots, zucchini or even canned and frozen varieties are great options.

Leftovers. If you plan to have leftovers you can have a meal ready to go for later in the week. This includes preparing more than you need for a meal and saving those extras. For example, if you are having a steak with vegetables on the side- you can cook double the amount of vegetables so that you have a "ready to eat" side item for a different dinner meal.

Freeze. Even foods such as chili and soup will be okay in the freezer. This is a great way to have smart food choices on hand for those times when you forgot to plan or just want something easy.

Delivery. This doesn't just mean ordering a pizza or take out. There are plenty of options now available for meal delivery services. Many of these will provide you with weekly meal plans where you get to experiment with recipes and ingredients that may be new to you. Intuitive eating shouldn't be limited to pre-planned meals, but this can be a great way to learn how to cook different meals or to have all the shopping done for you.

Themes. If you're trying to come up with ideas for your meal planning, you may want to consider having a "theme" night for one or more weekdays. For example, Taco Tuesdays or Pasta Wednesdays are an easy way to keep track of what you're going to cook throughout the week.

Remember, that meal planning for the intuitive eater is all about learning about the foods you like most and what preferences you have. In your journal make a sheet just for meal planning purposes. Come up with meal ideas, snack ideas, and ask yourself what you are in the mood for this week. Once you've got your list go through and ask yourself if those foods are things you like. Then consider which foods are "staple" items such as carbs, protein, fat, and fiber. Check your list to make sure these meal ideas provide you with foods that will be nourishing and satisfying.

Meal planning will look different for you from week to week depending on a variety of factors including your preferences, schedule, family, plans, etc. Give yourself permission to change up your meals that are planned if they no longer sound appealing when you're in the moment. You can always save something you had planned for later in the week!

CHAPTER 8:

CHPOOSING FOODS

Since intuitive eating has nothing to do with willpower, diets, or discipline choosing the best foods for our body can be a pleasant experience. You may already be drawn to certain foods, and you should continue to enjoy them when wanted. One of the main goals of intuitive eating is to allow ourselves to make better food choices so that we are providing the appropriate levels of nutrition.

There is a difference between feeling full and feeling satisfied. If we're out of touch with our bodies' needs it can be difficult to figure out what being comfortably full really feels like. Since the physical feeling of fullness usually isn't enough to stop us from eating, our satisfaction plays a large role. We can eat a full meal without feeling satisfied, and it can cause us to eat more food to fill that need even when we aren't hungry. Satisfaction is mainly mental sensation. We must work to find pleasure in the foods we eat so that we can feel both content and satisfied. A great place to start is to consider the foods that you enjoy and incorporate them into well-balanced meals that include fats, carbs, and protein.

The texture, smell, and taste of food contribute to the way we associate satisfaction we can get from it. This is a personal experience and will vary greatly for each person. This includes the perceived size of food. If we order a small diet focused meal we are less likely to feel as satisfied than if we order a king-size meal.

Fullness Factor

When we discuss the potential of certain foods to best keep us feeling full, we consider how satisfying they are per calorie. In general, those foods that are easy to overeat such as those with high amounts of sugar, fat and/or starch are the foods with the lowest fullness factor. Foods that have high amounts of water, fiber, and/or protein are those that have the highest potential to keep us full. Liquids are known for having high fullness factors, though for only short periods. This can be seen in foods like chips and candy bars being less likely to satiate our hunger while foods like watermelon and chicken breasts can go a long way in keeping us feeling full. Below are some foods that have the greatest potential for helping us to feel full.

Potatoes are one of those foods that are very filling and are known as a food with the highest satiety potential. Since they are high in carbohydrates and water they can help us feel full quickly and keep us from overeating. Potatoes contain a little bit of essentially every nutrient our bodies need!

Eggs are considered a "perfect" food because of the number of nutrients and protein in a low-calorie serving. They've even been shown to help people eat less for up to 36 hours after consuming them! The yolk of the egg is the most nutritious as they are loaded with protein, healthy fat, antioxidants and minerals.

Oatmeal is a great source of fiber while being low in calories. Because of their ability to soak up water, oats can go a long way in making us feel full. As a breakfast choice, it can help us consume fewer calories following the meal, and even delay the emptying of the stomach due to the way the high fiber content acts in the digestive system.

Fish is loaded with essential fats and high-quality protein. This can help to cause a stronger fullness effect than most other proteins. Not all fish is created equal. We want to consume fish that has a low level of contaminants, have high amounts of omega-3 fatty acids, and be raised/caught sustainably. Opt for mackerel, sardines, and salmon when possible.

Soup, although thought to be less filling than solid foods, can be very filling meals. It's been found that smooth soups last longer in the body and can prolong the feeling of fullness. Experiment with soup recipes that contain ingredients you like. Try adding a side of soup to a few of your meals during the week to help you feel full and to provide additional nutrients.

Meat is generally high in protein, and lean meats can satiate our hunger while providing a satisfying experience. While it's wise to limit the amount of high-fat red meat, incorporating meat into the diet can help us feel full-especially when consumed during the first half of the day.

Greek Yogurt is higher in protein than other varieties and can help us feel full until our next meal. Greek yogurt is different from most other yogurts because of the way that they whey is strained. This produces a creamier, thicker yogurt that is typically tarter. Be sure to find true Greek yogurt and not "Greek style" as those are typically made using thickening agents. Plenty of fat-free and sugar-free varieties are available, but they usually don't share the same health benefits. Greek Yogurt is rich in calcium and protein which can promote bone health as well as keep you feeling fuller longer. When we consume high-protein foods we can boost our metabolism as it increases the number of calories we burn each day. One of the most powerful benefits of Greek Yogurt is that it contains probiotics-or good bacteria that help restore a healthy balance within our gut.

Vegetables are loaded with all sorts of nutrients that our bodies require. They are high-volume foods with low-calorie content. In fact, one teaspoon of butter is the caloric equivalent of an entire half-cup of most vegetables! The amount of fiber and water that they contain adds bulk to our meals and can help to fill us up. In addition, they can take longer to fully chew, causing us to slow down in consuming our foods. Many of us were raised to "eat our vegetables" but it's common that we develop unhealthy associations with them. If we are something as a kid that we really didn't like, the chances are that we stay away from that food as an adult. The problem with this is that our taste buds mature as we do, and we could be avoiding something that we would enjoy.

Fruits contain high amounts of fiber and water which can provide the bulk needed to keep feelings of fullness longer. Juices may taste great but aren't very filling, so it's smart to opt for fresh fruits in their natural form. All fruits have antioxidants that combat free radicals. They can also help boost our brainpower and increase the functions of our digestive systems. Most fruits are packed with vitamins that are essential to proper functioning. Seek out grapefruit, mango, pineapple, grapes, berries, and citrus fruits when possible.

Nuts are energy-dense and full of nutrients. Because they are high in healthy fats and protein they can also be very filling. They've been shown to reduce hunger and provide essential fatty acids that our bodies require. They are naturally low in carbs and high in good fats as well as provide several nutrients and minerals. They are loaded with antioxidants and can even help lower our cholesterol and raise our "good" cholesterols. Nuts have been proven to provide anti-inflammatory effects, especially in those with serious health conditions.

Whole Grains are known to raise and lower our blood sugar much more slowly than high glycemic index foods. This can cause our hunger to be satiated for much longer periods while providing the fiber we need for healthy digestion. A whole grain is seeds of grass-like plants such as corn, rice, wheat, quinoa, amaranth, and buckwheat. A whole-grain kernel will include the bran, endosperm, and germ. If these three parts are present, it is considered a whole grain. They are loaded with fiber, vitamins and minerals, protein, and antioxidants. One of the best benefits of including whole grains in the diet is that they support a healthy digestive system. They are also known to reduce inflammation, reduce risk of cancers, as well as reduce risk for heart disease and strokes!

If you can incorporate some or all these foods into your daily nutrition, it can go a long way in increasing your overall health.

By choosing foods that help us to feel full and provide a satisfaction factor we can develop meal plans that we can go back to again and again. Choose nutrient-dense foods as much as you can.

Nutrient Density

Below is a list of some of most nutritious foods we can eat:

Fatty Fish. Salmon and other fatty fish are full of fatty acids, vitamins, protein, and minerals. Try to incorporate fatty fish in at least one meal a week.

Greens. Kale, Spinach, and Collards are just a few types of nutrient-dense green, leafy vegetables. These are some of the most nutritious foods you can eat as they contain high amounts of vitamins and minerals as well as fiber and protein. Greens also contain antioxidants and bioactive compounds that have cancer-fighting properties!

Garlic. High in vitamins and minerals, garlic also contains sulfur compounds that can help lower blood pressure and the risk of heart disease. Garlic consumption can also help fight cancer, and in its raw form it can be antibacterial and antifungal! Garlic is also easy to add to meals because its taste can enhance the flavor of most foods.

Blueberries. Most fruit is going to be a healthy choice, but blueberries are high in antioxidants proven to protect our brains and increase the level of antioxidants in our blood.

Dark Chocolate. Aside from tasting great, dark chocolate that has a high content of cocoa is one of the most nutrient-dense food options! Another powerhouse for antioxidants, cocoa can also help improve blood flow and lower blood pressure. The best will have 85% cocoa or higher.

The best way to get all the nutrients we need is by filling our meals with nutrient-dense foods such as those above. This doesn't mean replace what you are currently eating with only these foods. You can make easy, small shifts in your current diet to provide room for these nutritious choices. You can switch to brown or wild rice instead of white rice. You can try adding Greek yogurt to a bowl of chili instead of sour cream. You can snack on nuts or vegetables instead of chips. The food choices you make are going to directly impact the amount of energy and focus that you have.

CHAPTER 9:

EXERCISE

No matter where we are at on our journey to eating intuitively and living a healthier lifestyle, we can always benefit from simply moving our bodies. In fact, the more active we are the better our bodies can break down and use the nutrients we provide through the foods we eat! It is through exercise that our tissues receive oxygen and nutrients. It also helps our cardiovascular system to work more efficiently and increases our heart and lung capacity. Implementing a fitness program can be a very rewarding practice that can pay off in many ways. Not only will the physical activity reduce your risk for chronic disease, but it can also help relieve feelings of anxiety and depression, increase coordination and balance, and even help regulate our sleep patterns. You don't have to set up an exercise plan just to lose weight. You may already be at your ideal weight or want to maintain your current body mass. The best place to start is by taking a real assessment of your current fitness level. When you record basic fitness scores and measurements, it's not meant to judge or use to beat yourself up. You want to record your baseline scores so that you have benchmarks to use when measuring your progress. This goes beyond your weight. Focus on your aerobic and muscular fitness, your flexibility, body composition, and cardiovascular endurance. Here are a few measurements you may want to record before setting up your fitness plan:

Resting Heart Rate

Heart Rate after moderate, and extraneous activity (You can measure your heart rate before and after an activity)

How long it takes you to walk, and run 1 mile (if you can, measure both but if you cannot run 1 mile, measure how far you can run before needing to stop)

How many push-ups can you do at a time? (You can measure how many modified sit-ups you can do if needed)

With your legs in front of you while seated on the floor, measure how far you can reach

Standard measurements such as chest, waist, thighs, can be taken if you're interested in changing the measurements

Body Mass Index

Fitness Plan for the Intuitive Eater

Once you've decided to set up a fitness routine for yourself, you need to implement a plan. You'll want to consider the reasons for starting your fitness routine. When you can clearly define goals, it can help you to stay motivated and to gauge your progress. Maybe you want to increase your endurance so that you can run further without having to stop. Maybe you'd like to be able to perform 5 pull-ups. Maybe you're preparing for a marathon, or you simply want to be more active. You can tailor the activities you engage in to help you reach your goals. Studies have shown that we need around 150 minutes of moderate aerobic activity every week. You could substitute this for 75 minutes of vigorous aerobic activity or perform a combination of them. Ideally, you want to engage in at least 30 minutes of aerobic exercise every day, or as many days as you can. Incorporate strength training at least two days a week as well. Seek to create balance in your routine so that you're not becoming "burned out" by doing the same thing every day, or overexerting yourself.

If you have any mobility issues, injuries, or health-related issues, always consult your physician before participating in any physical activity. They can help you design a fitness program that's tailored to your individual needs and will improve your range of motion, endurance, and overall strength. When determining what activities to include in your fitness plan, consider those activities that you enjoy participating in. If you enjoy low-impact activities, seek out opportunities to bike or swim. Alternate these with strength training and you've got it worked out! If you enjoy the social aspects of going to the gym, find a group class to join! The more varied your activities are, the more interested you will be in continuing it. Sometimes it can help to write down your plan, and the activities that you want to participate in. You can use that to help stay on track, and to keep yourself motivated. Remember that if you haven't been working out regularly that you want to start out slowly and gradually build up your endurance. Many people will over-exert themselves during their first workout sessions and when it results in over-use of muscles and soreness or even injury, it can be very discouraging. Be sure that you are planning time between activities to rest and recover.

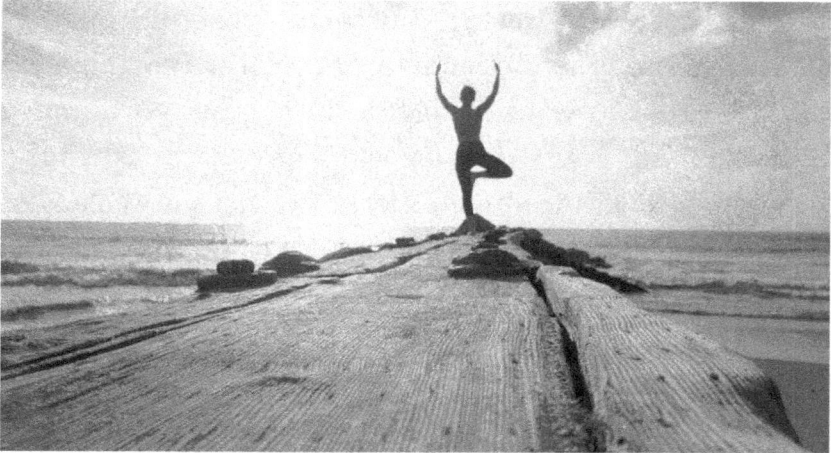

You will also want to consider using activity tracking apps so that you can focus on your activity while still getting accurate information on your progress. If you plan to purchase exercise equipment be sure to test it out to make sure that it's the right size and fits into your daily life. Find yourself a good pair of athletic shoes, as they will be the most important fitness equipment you will purchase. Remember that you don't have to perform all of your exercises at one time- you can engage in activities multiple times throughout the day. If you can't find 30-60 minutes a day, you may find that you can take 10-15 minutes multiple times a day and that will work just as well. Listen to your body and give yourself permission to take a day or two off if you're exhausted, sick, or simply don't want to. If you've taken a few days off and you don't have any motivation to continue with your fitness plan, you may want to reassess your reasons for doing it in the first place. After 6 weeks you'll want to retake your measurements and compare them with your starting results. Do this every few months so that you can compare your results with your efforts

Many of us have jobs where we are required to sit at a desk in front of a computer. Even those of us that have very active lifestyles outside of work are still impacted by the negative effects that sitting down for prolonged periods of time can cause. Studies have shown these effects include an increased risk for heart disease, cancers, and diabetes just to name a few! What's worse is that these effects aren't reversible through the activity we do outside of work. The only way to minimize these risks is to limit the amount of time we spend sitting throughout the day. The good news is that it can be easy to move our bodies during those work hours. Simply standing up frequently or taking a short walk once every couple of hours can go a long way.

Tips for being more active during the workday

Take the Stairs. We hear this all the time, but it really is a great way to increase the amount of physical activity you engage in without making a huge difference to your daily schedule. If you normally take the elevator, try taking it to one floor beneath your destination. Walk the one floor up the stairs.

Park further away. This is another easy way to increase the number of steps you are getting every day. This can be anywhere that you park your car; work, the grocery store, etc. We all have a habit of searching for the closest spot, but it's hardly ever because we are in a hurry. Parking in the back of the lot can also help to relieve any stress you feel when you can't find an ideal parking spot, because they are almost certainly always available.

Stand Up. If you have a sedentary desk job, it's important to limit the amount of time you stay in a seated position. There are huge health risks that are associated with sitting for long durations. We can work to mitigate those risks by simply standing up while we work. If you can stand at your desk, try to stand at least 15 minutes every hour.

Take a Walk. Even the most intense work schedules allow for a break. Take the long way when going to the restroom to get the extra steps in. Take the stairs and go to the restroom on a different floor if you are able. Try to take a short, brisk walk at least every few hours during the workday- even if it is just to the water-cooler.

Take your Lunch. It's important to give yourself enough time to enjoy your lunch break. If you have an active job where you are on your feet, take the time to relax and take the strain off your joints. If you have a sitting job, it can be helpful to prepare a lunch that doesn't take too long to eat so that you have some time to get outside and take a quick walk. If your company has an exercise room, you can always commit to using it a few times a week.

Stretch. Remember to stretch out your back and neck after long sessions of sitting. If you have an active job, remember to stretch before your shift and make time to stretch your back during the day. We want to ensure proper blood flow throughout the work day and stretching is a great way to relieve built-up tension in our bodies.

Participate. Many employers offer fitness groups or classes that you can join. A simple yoga class or pilates session can really help to fit in exercise during an otherwise busy day.

There are lots of different ways that we can be more active during the day. This includes weekends. If you find yourself catching up on sleep during the weekends, try to work in time for exercise before or after. It's by making a commitment to be active whenever you can that will really help in the long run. Exercise doesn't have to be something you dread, and it can even turn into something you look forward to once you discover those activities you truly enjoy!

CHAPTER 10:

TRACKING PROGRESS

Most of the time when we are tracking our progress when it comes to eating, we are doing so with a dieting mindset. Since eating intuitively isn't measured by the pounds we lose or the inches that are shed, it can be hard to measure the progress that we are making. In your food journal, you can keep track of the meals you are eating and the foods that are bringing you the greatest feelings of fullness and satisfaction. There are many ways that we can measure the progress that do not include a scale or the number of calories we consume. You may want to take a few "before" photos, especially if your goal is to lose weight or increase physical activity. While we may not notice changes or progress in looking in the mirror every day, we can easily see changes in photos taken once a month or so. Keep in mind that we are always improving, and there really isn't going to be a "before" and "after" like there would be in dieting gimmicks. Keeping track of how your skin looks is a great way to see progress. If you are moving your body and sweating out toxins, it can help to detoxify your body and lead to improved skin.

Try to create a plan to track your progress. You may want to set "check-in" points such as 30, 60, and 90-day timeframes.

After that, you can continue to track on a monthly, quarterly, or bi-annual basis.

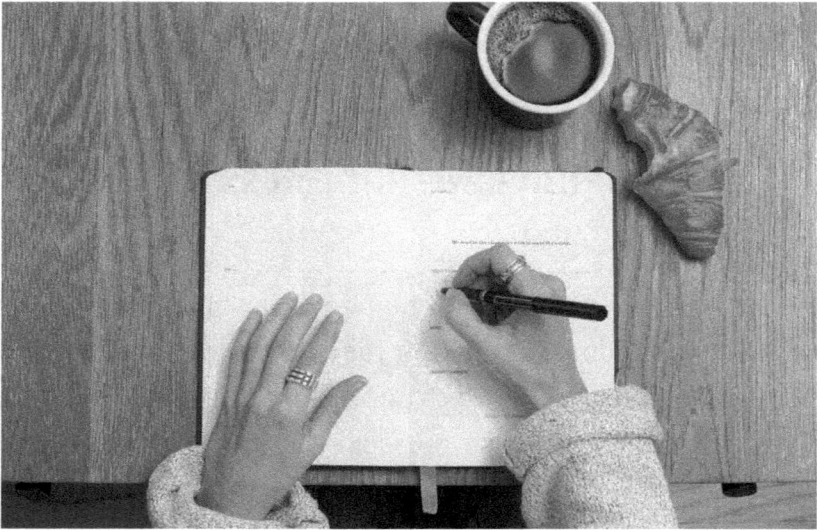

What to Track

Here are some ideas to help you measure your progress with intuitive eating:

Hunger Cues

Are you able to notice when you are feeling physical hunger? Are you honoring that hunger by feeding it? By trusting your body when it lets you know it's hungry-even at odd hours, or after you've already eaten something is important to your progress. When first starting out, you'll want to assess how likely you are to recognize physical hunger from mental hunger. After a period of a few months, how has this improved? In what ways?

Fullness

When first starting out, we might not be able to tell when we are full. You may not know which foods provide that feeling for you, or how much you need to eat before you reach satisfaction. Take a baseline measurement of this with certain foods or meals and compare them to how you measure up a few months into intuitive eating. As yourself how often you finish a meal and still aren't satisfied. Also, examine how often you are eating to excess simply because the food is good. Tracking your fullness is all about rediscovering your body's natural signal that you've had enough and listening to it.

Stress

How much do you currently stress about the foods you eat? Do you find yourself thinking about what you're going to eat and how much you'll have instead of enjoying your food? We can measure our progress when it comes to stressing less about food. Notice the ways that you are exerting your control over food.

Satisfaction

When beginning to eat intuitively, you may not really know which foods are satisfying and which ones are not. This should encourage you to play around with the foods you enjoy and prepare them in different ways. When you find foods that are satisfying and keep you feeling full. Make note of them. Measure the difference from how many foods you can describe as being satisfying to how many you can name in 3 months.

Mindfulness

In what ways are you currently being distracted during mealtimes? Make a list of all the ways that distractions can be keeping you from eating intuitively and recognizing your hunger and fullness symptoms. Keep track of ways that you can be more mindful. Make note of how your favorite foods smell, taste, and feel. Attempt to slow down and keep track of how often you are pausing before you eat.

Variety

Are you currently eating a wide variety of foods? Do you have certain foods that you've picked up from dieting that you consider "safe" or "good"? You can measure your progress by incorporating those foods that you may have considered off-limits or bad. Keep track of those foods that you are staying away from now, and which ones you discover as enjoyable along the way.

Emotional Health

If you have identified certain triggers that lead you to emotional eating, you can measure the ways that change this behavior. Maybe you list out different coping mechanisms that you can employ when you feel triggered. You can keep track of how effective something is or is not for you.

Energy

With intuitive eating, you will become more in tune with your body and the foods that help you feel your best. Make note of when you have the most energy during the day, and what foods help with your energy levels and which ones don't. You can track those foods that keep you fueled, and what you can rely on when you need an energy boost.

Stopping Ability

When you begin to eat more mindfully and take the time to truly taste and enjoy your food, you are more able to recognize when something isn't enjoyable for you and make the decision to stop eating it. This can be hard or those "waste-not" eaters that feel they must clean their plates at every meal. The ability to stop mid-meal because you've learned that you don't enjoy something can be just as powerful as any other method. You can track this by your current ability to stop, and how that's changed over the course of a couple of months.

Exercise

Measuring your progress when it comes to exercise can be easy, and fun. Take a few baseline measurements such as how many push-ups, sit-ups, and jumping jacks you can do. After a 90-day commitment to simply moving your body every day, take those measurements again. Notice what's changed, and what you'd like to improve upon further. This can be applied to any of the ways that you enjoy moving your body. Feel free to set a goal for yourself such as a 30-day squat or push-up challenge. Compare your results after the 30 days to see how far you've come!

Consider your current body image and the ways you view

your self-worth. You'll be putting in a lot of work in the coming months with getting to know yourself and accepting your body for what it does for you. As you continue your journey, you will notice an increase in your confidence. This confidence can affect the way you view yourself, and how others see you as well. Measure where you think you are on a scale of 1-10 when it comes to the ways you see yourself and take that assessment again in a few months.

Remember to set goals for yourself that are attainable. If you want to be more active, then commit to going for a walk once a week. Once you achieve that goal, set it to twice a week, and so on. When you are tracking your progress with intuitive eating, you want to consider how you feel. Since there is no structure in how or when you are eating your meals, you'll have to determine what is right for you personally. Stop comparing yourself to others and what they are eating. Each of us will have completely different experiences with food.

You'll want to consider your ideal relationship with food. Since there is no end to intuitive eating, this is important. Every time we eat, we should be doing so in response to a cue from our body. When you can trust yourself to make the right decisions regarding what you eat, and when you stop eating- you will be well on your way to having a strong mind/body connection. Some days will be harder than others, and most time you'll listen to your body without really thinking about it. This is something that we do naturally, and when we can separate ourselves from the dieting culture, we can reconnect to those natural tendencies we all have.

CONCLUSION

Thank you for making it through to the end of *Intuitive Eating Workbook: A step by step mindful program for weight loss,* let's hope it was informative and able to provide you with all the tools you need to achieve your goals whatever they may be.

The next step is to begin by using this workbook on your journey to eating intuitively. This means taking an honest assessment of where you are currently when it comes to your relationship to food and eating. Developing a healthy relationship with food and strengthening your mind-body connection are the key goals of intuitive eating. If you're coming from a diet mindset, this can be difficult as you probably have habits of restricting your food intake and worrying over calories and what the scales say. Identifying what type of eater you are, and what different emotions could be driving your eating decisions is a powerful way to recognize how your current relationship to food compares to how you would like for it to be. Reflect on your food journal every week, and eventually, it will become a natural habit to consider how your meals tasted, and if they were satisfying.

Use this workbook to help you identify the ways that you use food to soothe yourself when experiencing different emotions. Really ask yourself what foods you consider off-limits, and what you're keeping yourself from enjoying. Many of us have years of experience with fad diets and weight loss tactics, but very little experience when it comes to really recognizing when we are hungry. Knowing the difference between physical and emotional hunger is one of the most important aspects of intuitive eating. Take the time to discover your personal triggers and the foods that they cause you to reach for. Once you've done this you can start to make smart decisions when it comes to nutrition. Be sure to incorporate nutrient-dense foods as many times during the week as you can.

Intuitive eating is the anti-diet, and it can take some time to remove those habits that are ingrained in each of us when it comes to weight loss and portion control. Discovering the foods that help you feel not only full but also satisfied can help you develop your own personal nutrition plan. Since no foods are off-limits, you can really explore different tastes and preferences that you may not be familiar with. Practice mindful eating by eating slowly, sitting down to eat, and really focusing on how foods make you feel. Create a nutritionally balanced meal plan that includes fresh fruits and vegetables, carbohydrates, healthy fats, and lean proteins. Determine your hunger scale, and honor that hunger. If you're hungry, eat! When you're full, stop!

Use intuitive eating to help you reach your fitness and nutrition goals. No matter your current relationship with food, you can easily set and attain your goals with a little focus and determination.

CPSIA information can be obtained
at www.ICGtesting.com
Printed in the USA
LVHW051944010421
683231LV00016B/703

9 781801 321099